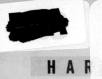
What is . . .

STRESS?

To a musician the word *stress* can mean to emphasize a particular note. To a linguist it means emphasizing a particular word. To a biologist *stress* means anything that constitutes a real or apparent threat to an organism. A surgeon uses the word *stress* to describe a kind of fracture. But most of us will use the word *stress* as a way of saying that we feel tired, pressurized, exhausted, unhappy, overworked, tense, powerless, fearful—or distressed.

There are many different kinds of stress . . .

Stress is not all bad . . .

Stress can never be avoided . . .

But it *can* be controlled!

Other HarperEssentials

FIRST AID
UNDERSTANDING DREAMS
WINE GUIDE

HARPERESSENTIALS

Stress Survival Guide

Jit Gill

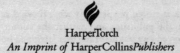

HarperTorch
An Imprint of HarperCollins*Publishers*

This title was first published by HarperCollins UK in 1999.

Illustrations by David Mostyn

Many thanks to Hodder and Stoughton publishers for permission to reproduce the quizzes: Are You a Type A Personality?, pp.17–20 and How Well Do You Cope With Stress?, pp. 35–38. These are taken from *Managing Stress* by Terry Looker and Olga Gregson.

HARPERTORCH
An Imprint of HarperCollins*Publishers*
10 East 53rd Street
New York, New York 10022-5299

Copyright © Grapevine Publishing Services Ltd, 1999
ISBN: 0-06-053454-0

First HarperTorch paperback printing: August 2003

HarperCollins ®, HarperTorch™, and ♥™ are trademarks of Harper-Collins Publishers Inc.

Printed in the United States of America

Visit HarperTorch on the World Wide Web at www.harpercollins.com

10 9 8 7 6 5 4 3 2 1

Contents

CONTENTS

CONTENTS

CONTENTS

Introduction

The word "stress" is a modern one—a catch-all term used to describe a variety of emotions and experiences. Where once we may have said that we felt worried, nervous, tense, unhappy or panicky, today we increasingly say that we feel stressed. We use "stress" to explain the kind of day we've had; we use it when we've had a run-in with the boss; we use it when we have had an argument with our children; and we use it when describing yet another disastrous journey on public transportation.

The all-encompassing usage of the word is partly

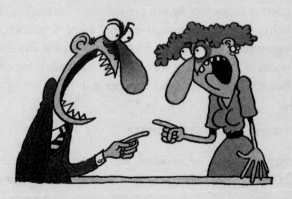

what makes stress so hard to pin down or recognize in practical terms. Also, stress affects everyone differently. An event that might send one person's blood pressure through the roof, will leave another untouched.

Part of the problem of dealing with stress is familiarity. We have become so used to living with stress, in its many guises—fatigue, overwork, moving, changing jobs, grief—that we may not fully realize how deeply it can influence our lives. Stress affects not only our emotional wellbeing but our physical health too.

STRESS IS NOT ALL BAD

It's wrong to think of stress as a dark predatory force to be avoided at all costs. It's not. Each and every one of us experiences some stress in our lives. And for good reasons too. Stress provides the adrenaline that helps to get us through exams, meet deadlines, or move to a new home. In this way stress can be a positive, motivating force which can work for us— boosting our health and wellbeing.

THERE'S NO ESCAPE FROM STRESS

Stress cannot be avoided, but it can be controlled. Learning how to manage stress is key to whether it becomes a friend or foe. More often than not, it's not the stressful event but our response to it that causes all the trouble. Time and again, research has shown that changing our response to stress helps to transform it from a negative to a positive experience, releasing unknown energy reserves, which help us to lead happier and more fulfilled lives.

WHAT IS STRESS?

Stress is hard to define and answers will vary depending on who you speak to. To a musician the word stress can mean to emphasize a particular note. To a linguist it means emphasizing a particular word. To a biologist stress means anything that constitutes a real or apparent threat to an organism. A surgeon uses the word stress to describe a kind of fracture. But most of us will use the word stress as a way of saying that we feel tired, pressurized, exhausted, unhappy, overworked, tense, powerless or fearful—or distressed.

And there are many different types of stress.

EMOTIONAL AND MENTAL STRESS

This can be caused by:

- work problems
- relationship difficulties

- money worries
- taking tests or going for job interviews

Signs of emotional and mental stress may include:

- anger
- jealousy
- fear
- worry
- depression
- low self-esteem
- poor concentration
- inability to make decisions

PHYSICAL AND ENVIRONMENTAL STRESS

This form of stress tends to be overshadowed by emotional stress, but it must not be overlooked as it can be just as detrimental to our health.

Physical/environmental stress may be caused by:

- over-exercising—training too long or too hard
- strenuous physical labor, such as carrying too many heavy objects

- traumatic jolting, such as a whiplash injury sustained in a car accident
- going through extreme temperature changes

Signs of physical and environmental stress may include:

- muscular aches and pains
- poor posture
- puffy eyes
- dehydrated skin

A VICIOUS CYCLE

Whether your stress is emotional and/or mental, or physical and/or environmental in origin, one often leads to another: emotional or mental stress invariably leads to physical stress, and extreme physical stress can affect your emotional and mental wellbeing.

This can set up a vicious cycle, especially in people with long-term or chronic stress, making it even harder to resolve the problem.

WHAT TRIGGERS STRESS?

When we talk about feeling stressed, we tend to use it in terms of the event that left us feeling stressful, but this is more correctly known as a stressor.

A stressor can range from a major life experience (divorce, bereavement, job loss or moving to a new house) to minor everyday annoyances.

WHAT HAPPENS TO OUR BODIES?

Dr. Hans Selye, the authority on stress, defines it as "the rate of wear and tear on the body." He showed that whatever the cause of the stress—cold, heat, anger, pain, grief or even happiness—the same physiological response occurs in our bodies. Selye called this the General Adaptation Syndrome. It is also known as the stress response or stress reaction. There are three stages to this syndrome:

1. The alarm stage
2. The resistance stage
3. Exhaustion

THE ALARM STAGE

Dr. Selye also called this stage the "fight or flight" response. This is our initial response to danger or a threat and is designed to help us cope with a crisis. It can be traced back to early on in our evolution, where survival meant being able to outrun or overpower predators. This is a positive response which provides the body with a rush of energy and power that increases our physical and mental capabilities.

For our ancestors, the alarm stage would have been triggered by the appearance of a saber-toothed

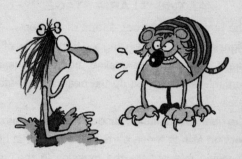

tiger looking for lunch. Today, the sight of a car heading straight for us, an argument or confrontation, suddenly remembering we didn't switch the iron off when we left the house, preparing to take a driving test, or rushing to catch an airplane, will all set off this reaction.

In modern life, however, it is not always appropriate to deal with stress on such a basic level. Hitting your boss is not always the best way to ensure that your needs are met. But running away from stress is not always the solution either. So instead we bottle up our feelings, and with no clear outlet for the physical and emotional effects of the adrenaline being pumped around our body, the stressed-out feeling remains. In the long term this can affect our health.

WHAT HAPPENS TO THE BODY AT THE "ALARM STAGE"?

- The brain perceives some form of danger.
- Signals from the brain trigger the release of the stress hormones—adrenaline, noradrenaline and cortisol—which speed up the heart and breathing rates.
- The heart beats faster. Blood is diverted from the gut and skin to those parts of the body that need to swing into action—the muscles in the trunk, arms and legs.
- Kidney function slows because there is less blood available for it to do its work.
- The muscles contract ready for sudden movement.
- The pupils of the eyes dilate.
- The salivary glands dry up and the mouth feels dry.
- Skin may turn pale as surface blood vessels contract to divert more blood to the muscles.
- Sweating increases and you may feel hot and bothered.
- The lungs must take in more air to supply more oxygen needed for energy to the muscles, but at the same time they must also get rid of more car-

bon dioxide, so breathing becomes quicker or deeper.

• The liver releases more sugar and fat to provide energy for the muscles.

• Digestion slows or stops and the sphincter muscles close up to avoid defecation and urination. Sometimes the opposite can happen which is where we get the phrase "wetting your pants with fear," or diarrhea can occur.

All these, plus other complex changes, can take place in an instant.

THE RESISTANCE STAGE

The alarm reaction does not last for very long. But many stressors continue long after the fight or flight response has worn off. In the resistance stage the amount of adrenaline in the blood decreases and different hormones swing into action to help the body adapt and deal with prolonged stress. These include cortisol which increases blood-sugar levels to give the body much needed energy, and aldosterone which helps to keep the blood pressure raised under long periods of stress, enabling the body to carry out important circulatory tasks.

EXHAUSTION

This happens when we no longer have the resources to deal with prolonged stress. The first two stages in the General Adaptation Syndrome are designed to be short-lived. We perceive a danger and respond to it, and once some kind of physical action has been taken (we have either fought or fled), the danger has passed and the stress hormones flooding our body have been used as nature intended, we can relax.

Although stage two allows us to cope with prolonged stress, it does not do so indefinitely. If we do not allow ourselves to recuperate but keep on pushing ourselves to handle the stress, the time will come when we will simply no longer be able to marshal the resources needed to deal with a situation. When this happens the body collapses or burns out, and illness or even death can result.

HORMONES DON'T LAST FOREVER

Our stress hormones not only produce the stress reaction; they also help us tolerate prolonged stress. But our supply of them is limited. And our body constantly has to produce them from "scratch," from the food we eat, to replace those used up during stress.

If there are not enough nutrients in the body to make fresh supplies or if we are using them more quickly than we make them, we simply run out. This is known as adrenal exhaustion. When this happens our stress tolerance decreases and we find it hard to cope with even mildly stressful situations. Blood-sugar levels are also reduced, so there is less energy going to the brain and other muscles in the body which can result in chronic fatigue.

GOOD STRESS V. BAD STRESS

Dr. Hans Selye distinguished between good and bad stress. A certain amount of good stress, sometimes called "eustress," can be good for us. Good stress is a positive force that stretches us and keeps us on our toes. We all need a certain amount of stimulation to motivate and spice up our lives, to allow us to take on new challenges and opportunities, and to meet our goals. Eustress is the "buzzy" feeling that helps us to meet urgent deadlines or get a complicated dinner party menu ready on time. Without this our lives would be dull and boring.

But there is a fine line between good stress and bad stress. As with so many other parts of life, you can get too much of a good thing, and good stress will surely lead to distress if you allow it to get out of control. This, in turn, can have a devastating effect on your life.

Bad stress is by no means confined to the high-fliers with busy jobs and even busier lives. People with too much free time and not enough to occupy their energy experience stress just as much as those who are rushed off their feet.

A LITTLE STRESS IS GOOD FOR US

Some of the hormones released in the body in stressful situations, such as adrenaline, also stimulate the immune system. In this way short-term stress can speed up the body's healing process. Long-term stress, however, depletes our body's supply of stress hormones, weakens the immune system and leaves us more vulnerable to disease.

Who is Most Likely to Suffer from Stress?

In an attempt to define who reacts well to stress and why, researchers have developed various classifications of personality types, described in this section: hot/cool, introvert/extrovert and Type A/Type B.

Where one person may fret over whether or not they can afford to buy something new to wear at the office Christmas party, another will just splash out and not give the expense a second thought. American stress experts call these two types "hot" and "cool" reactors.

- **Hot reactors** respond to unfamiliar situations as if they are threatening. Even just thinking that an event could be stressful, they will trigger a fight or flight response. As a result they will feel fearful, overstretched, anxious or angry for much of the time, so putting their bodies under a huge amount of stress. Hot reactors can, however, teach themselves to stay calm.

◉ **Cool reactors** take all that life has to throw at them in their stride. They are sometimes said to have a "hardy" or "stress-resistant" personality. These people are characterized by the "three Cs": Commitment, Control and Challenge:

> Commitment to all areas of their life: work, themselves, their job, their family and community
> Control: they have a sense of purpose and direction in their life and believe that they can influence events.
> Challenge: they see changes in life as normal and positive, and view them as a normal part of life rather than a threat.

Not everyone arrives in the world with these traits, but they can be learned.

GENES OR ENVIRONMENT

Our upbringing and life experiences partly determine our attitude and opinions. But certain basic traits are believed to be inherited. When shown a glass that is half filled with water there are those that will say it is half empty, and others who will say it is half full. This world view reflects whether you are optimistic or pessimistic. You can also inherit other traits:

whether you are tidy or untidy, organized or chaotic, introverted or extroverted.

Some stress experts believe that our genes can influence the way we respond to stress in just the same way that one family may be prone to digestive problems and another to eczema.

The kind of personality we have also determines the kind of stress we experience.

- **Introverts and pessimists** are most prone to chronic, insidious stress such as loneliness. This type of stress hones in on the immune system (the body's protection against disease), so that colds or infections are easily picked up.
- **Extroverts and highly organized control freaks** rarely stop to catch their breath and by doing so they too place a huge burden on their body's immune system. Like the introvert they are also more likely to pick up colds and viruses than those who take life at a slower more relaxed pace, who set aside time to relax rather than stretching themselves to the limit trying to get everything done.

Feeling angry and hostile to those around you will also determine how you respond to stress. When we are angry our body produces more of the stress hormones adrenaline and noradrenaline. In the long term this reduces our body's ability to fight disease, and can cause high blood pressure and heart disease.

Some stress researchers divide people into personality types according to how they respond to stressful situations, with A and B being the two main categories.

TYPE A PERSONALITIES

In the 1960s it was believed that workaholics with hair-trigger tempers and aggressive natures were more prone to heart disease. This group became known as the Type A personalities. But not all Type As are prone to heart disease. Some stress researchers, such as Dr. Redford Williams, a behavioural medicine researcher at Duke University in North Carolina, deny claims that all people with a Type A personality are at a higher risk of suffering a heart attack. For Dr. Williams, it's not the enthusiastic doers who are in danger but those who have a hostile attitude. Other researchers, such as Suzanne Kobasa of City University of New York, believe that Type As have a certain level of hardiness or stress resistance that helps to protect them from health problems.

So Type As can be subdivided into the hostile Type As and the hardy Type As.

Hostile Type As tend to be fairly isolated because people avoid their company. They can be slightly

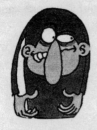

paranoid, believing that everyone is trying to trip them up in some way.

The defining feature of hardy Type As is that they regard situations as challenges rather than threats. They believe that change is good, are committed to what they do and feel confident about their ability to control their lives. Hardy Type As are able to keep stress in perspective and tend to have good interpersonal relationships.

Having plenty of friends you can share your worries with and a lively social life seems to lessen the impact of stress, say the researchers.

ARE YOU A TYPE A PERSONALITY?

This assessment of your level of Type A behavior can only be as accurate as you are honest in your answers. The problem is that Type As are often blind to their own behavior: the fact that they do everything very quickly, for example. The questionnaire is based on some common Type A characteristics, many of which are easy to spot, while others are more subtle. If a person has a large number of Type A characteristics and exhibits them frequently and excessively then he or she is considered to be an extreme Type A.

Give yourself a score of 0–5 for your answers as follows:

5 = always
4 = almost always
3 = usually
2 = sometimes
1 = almost never
0 = never

● Are you competitive in the games you play at home or at work?

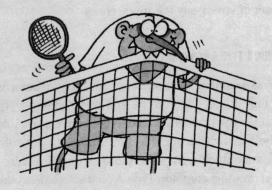

● Are you late for appointments?
● In conversation do you anticipate what others are going to say, nod your head, interrupt or finish sentences for them?

- Do you have to do things in a hurry?
- Do you get impatient waiting in lines or traffic jams?
- Do you try to do several things at once and think about what you are about to do next?
- Do you feel that you do most things quickly— eating, walking, talking, driving?
- Do you get easily irritated over trivia?
- If you make a mistake, do you get angry with yourself?
- Do you find fault with and criticize other people?

How to score: Total your score and multiply it by two.

Type B: 0–39

You are slightly and/or rarely impatient and aggravated. You create almost no unnecessary stress for yourself at all, and your health is probably unaffected.

Mild Type A: 40–59

You are fairly and/or occasionally impatient and aggravated. You create some unnecessary stress for yourself and this may affect your health.

Moderate Type A: 60–79

You are very and/or often impatient and aggravated.

You generate much unnecessary stress for yourself and this may affect your health.

Extreme Type A: 80–100

You are extremely and/or usually impatient and aggravated. You generate too much unnecessary stress for yourself and this may affect your health.

HOW TO SPOT TYPE A BEHAVIOR

In an attempt to gain control, Type As adopt two strategies to help them save time and achieve more:

- To squeeze more and more out of their day, Type As will try to get things done quicker to save time. They eat, walk, drive and talk fast.
- Type As practice polyphasing, which means doing two or more things at the same time. Some Type A men will shave while eating breakfast or use two electric razors to save time, while some Type A

women blow-dry their hair with two hair-driers for the same reason. Type As will brush their teeth or shave while taking a shower or continue writing a document while speaking on the telephone about a completely different subject.

- In the supermarket a Type A shopper approaching the check-out will make a number of decisions before choosing a line. They will typically count the number of people waiting, then quickly multiply this by the number of items in each shopping cart. A Type A will also estimate the efficiency of the person at the checkout. With all this data the Type A will join the "fastest" line. But instead of waiting patiently, the Type As watch the progression of the other lines to work out if they made the right choice. Their stress-hormone levels begin to rise when they see that the other lines are moving faster. They almost hit the roof when their line is held up by someone having to get a price checked, and they explode when it's their turn at last and the receipt roll runs out!

STRESS ADDICTION

While a Type A person will say that they thrive on stress, the reality is that they are addicted to the feelings of elation and confidence that a surge of noradrenaline creates.

Signs that you could be hooked on noradrenaline:

- your mind frequently races
- you experience disturbed sleep
- you smoke too much
- you drink excess caffeine
- you are hyperactive

⦿ Type As are prone to workaholism. As they strive for success and work longer and longer hours to achieve their aims, Type As typically experience marital and social problems. They find it difficult to relax, to switch off from work, and often take work home.

TYPE B PERSONALITIES

If you scored less than 40 in the quiz on pp. 18–19, you are probably a Type B personality. Although they are not as driven as Type As, this does not mean that Type Bs are less ambitious or successful. It's just that their approach is very different. In the long run they are often more effective than Type As because they don't panic, lose their temper or operate on high anxiety levels. They are good at giving attention to different areas of their life, such as their families and friends, and may have a creative outlet as well.

LIFE SKILLS

Your ability to cope with stress also depends on how well prepared you are to deal with and maintain a balance between the everyday demands that life throws at you. People with poor coping skills feel that they are constantly at the mercy of uncontrollable, unforeseen demands. Some people appear to be born with good coping skills, but they can be learned and improved upon. They include:

- assertiveness
- rational thinking
- organization
- quality of relationships
- quantity of relationships
- looking after yourself

THE T-TYPE PERSONALITY

Stress researchers have also identified another type of personality—the thrill-seeker or risk-taker. You can spot this personality a mile away. They seek out the challenges that others would never contemplate, such as parachuting or hang-gliding. They are the extroverts of any group and they are incredibly resilient to stress.

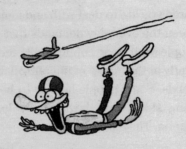

How Do You Know You Are Stressed?

For some people stress is so much a part of their life, that they may not even recognize the huge strain they are living under. They may be in a constant state of arousal, their bodies sending out whole armies of stress hormones to deal with the never-ending flow of crises, so that they never get a chance to return to normal and stabilize.

When there is an imbalance between the demands of everyday life and your ability to cope, you are likely to develop physical or emotional signs of stress. These are a signal that our stress resources are running out and it's time to act. The heavier and more prolonged your stress load and the less you feel able to deal with it, the more serious your symptoms are likely to be.

Below are lists of all the physical and emotional symptoms of excessive stress.

Do you suffer from:

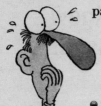

- aches and pains, particularly back and chest pains
  - palpitations
    - fainting or dizzy spells
  - sweating
  - poor appetite
  - food cravings
- indigestion, heartburn or stomach aches
- nervous twitching
- stammering
- nausea
- diarrhea, constipation or frequent urination
- headaches
- insomnia
- breathlessness without exertion
- hyperventilation
- constant tiredness
- constant colds and infections
- impotence or frigidity

Do you often feel:

- depressed
- irritable
- lethargic or exhausted
- unable to cope
- unable to concentrate
- as if you are constantly running out of time

- so angry you want to scream
- anxious for no apparent reason
- worried over minor things
- panicky about everyday events
- a failure
- inadequate
- that you jump from task to task without finishing anything
- unable to sit still
- afraid of being alone
- bored with work or home life
- disinterested in sex
- dissatisfied with life, but unsure why
- that you want to cry over "nothing"
- unable to make decisions
- that your memory is failing
- unable to talk to people
- that you want to run away
- unable to laugh

Do you:
- find it hard to relax
- bite your nails
- drink too much alcohol
- smoke heavily
- drink excessive amounts of coffee and tea
- take tranquilizers or other drugs
- suffer from phobias or obsessions

- worry about falling ill
- no longer feel bothered about personal hygiene or taking care of your appearance

If you frequently experience any of the above or can't remember a time when you didn't, then it is time to take action. Take up some of the suggestions in this book. You would also be advised to visit your doctor, as some of the complaints listed can also be a sign of physical or mental illness. Ignore them at your peril!

STRESSORS

The causes of stress are known as "stressors." These are life events or situations that can send our blood pressure soaring. Stressors can be directly threatening events such as being mugged or having a serious accident, or everyday occurrences with some kind of change involved. Change is stressful as it can often mean ending familiar routines and getting used to new ones.

In the 1960s two American scientists Dr. Thomas Holmes and Dr. Richard Rahe formally rated the effects that different life events could have on our lives. They developed what they called a "Social Readjustment Rating" which is also known as "the Stress Chart." Points were allocated on a scale of 1 to

100 to major life events such as divorce or marriage. By adding up the life events experienced by one person in a year, it is possible, in theory, to work out their chances of developing a stress-related illness.

Although the Stress Chart was devised some years ago it is still a useful method of assessing the possible stress implications of different life changes and events.

CHECK YOUR LIFE-EVENT STRESS

The following list will give you an idea of how stressful certain life events are. The higher the score the more stressful the event. Simply check off those life events you have experienced in the past year. A score of over 150 indicates a 50-percent chance of developing a stress-related illness in the near future. A score of more than 300 raises that likelihood to 90 percent.

Death of a spouse or partner	100
Divorce	73
Marital separation	65
Serving a jail sentence	63
Death of a close relative	63
Serious illness or injury	53
Marriage	50
Loss of job	47
Marital reconciliation	45

Retirement	45
Change in family member's health	44
Pregnancy	40
Sexual difficulties	39
New baby or family member	39
Significant change to financial status[1]	37
Death of a close friend	36
Change in line of work	35
Increase in domestic arguments	35
Large mortgage	31
Foreclosure of mortgage or loan	30
More or less responsibility at work	29
Child leaving home	29
Friction with in-laws	29
Outstanding personal achievement	28
Spouse starting or ending work	26
Starting or completing education	26
Change in living conditions	25
Change in personal habits	24
Trouble with employer	23
Change in working hours or conditions	20
Moving house	20
Changing school	20
Change in recreation	20
Change in church activities[2]	19
Change in social life	19

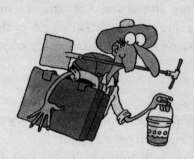

Notes

[1] Gaining a lot of money will place a different kind of pressure on someone than losing a lot, but it is nevertheless a significant cause of stress.

[2] This could mean taking up a new religious faith or changing your beliefs.

[3] This covers family rifts or arguments, as well as gaining new members of the family through marriage, so that there is a new line-up at family events.

CHECK YOUR STRESS RATING

As we've seen, any kind of change can be stressful but different people respond to stress in different ways.

The following questionnaire will help you to work out how the stresses and strains of everyday life affect you. For each question jot down the number which best represents the frequency of your symptoms:

1 = never
2 = infrequently: more than once every six months but less than once a month
3 = occasionally: more than once a month but less than once a week
4 = very often, more than once a week
5 = constantly

Then add up your score and read the "Understanding your score" panel (pp 33–5).

Emotional symptoms

1. Do you find it easy to relax? ❑
2. Do you get angry very easily? ❑
3. Do you frequently get bored? ❑
4. Do you find it hard to concentrate? ❑
5. Do you have anxious thoughts? ❑

6. Do you ever find it hard to make decisions? ❏
7. Do you feel frustrated? ❏
8. Do you feel hostile? ❏
9. Are you ever impatient? ❏
10. Do you experience racing thoughts? ❏
11. Do you have difficulty sleeping? ❏

Physical symptoms

1. Do you get headaches? ❏
2. Do you ever feel your heart pounding? ❏
3. Do you ever have allergic reactions? ❏
4. Do you suffer from indigestion? ❏
5. Do you grind your teeth? ❏
6. Do you suffer from neckache? ❏
7. Do you ever feel exhausted? ❏
8. Do you suffer from backache? ❏
9. Do your hands or feet feel sweaty? ❏
10. Do you get stomach aches? ❏
11. Do you find yourself trembling? ❏
12. Do you ever get a feeling of tightness in
    your chest? ❏
13. Are you unable to control your emotions? ❏

UNDERSTANDING YOUR SCORE

Under 60: You have low psychological and physical symptoms of stress. You cope well with whatever stress you come up against. Note, however, that this analysis refers only to your present stress level, so don't rest on your laurels: something could happen next week that would show a very different picture if you took the test again.

Remember also that being under-stressed can be just as problematic as being over-stressed. Symptoms include lethargy and boredom. If this sounds like you, aim to keep your body and mind stimulated. Do some exercise, take on new challenges and think positive.

61–80: You are showing moderate psychological and physical stress symptoms. You are not in the danger zone yet, but you could be if you are not careful. If you scored a five in one or two symptom areas, you could be holding on to a past stress. Unresolved issues and unsettled business, which happened years ago can cause just as much stress as present-day factors. If this sounds like you, try to identify and address the problem. If you feel unable to deal with it, you many find it useful to see a holistic practitioner, doctor or counselor.

81–100: You are showing high psychological and physical stress symptoms. You need to act now.

Follow the instant and long-term stress-busting plans carefully (see pp. 197–231). Do some of the relaxation exercises daily and focus on the issues that are causing you problems, dealing with them one at a time.

100: You have excessive psychological and physical stress symptoms. You are heading towards psychological and physical burnout. If you don't act now to improve your lifestyle you could be on the way to a full nervous breakdown. Act now to beat long-term and short-term stress or seek professional help.

HOW WELL DO YOU COPE WITH STRESS?

Managing stress effectively is a question of keeping it in balance. This can be done either by altering the demands being made on you or by improving your ability to cope with them.

Complete the questionnaire below with "Yes" or "No" answers to find out how you currently cope with stress.

PART 1

1. Do you have supportive family and friends? ❏
2. Do you have a hobby? ❏
3. Do you belong to a social or activity group? ❏
4. Do you practice any relaxation techniques (such as yoga, meditation, creative imagery, autogenic training) on a daily basis? ❏
5. Do you exercise for at least 20 minutes three times a week? ❏

6. Do you do something just for yourself each week that you really enjoy? ❏
7. Do you have somewhere you can go to be alone? ❏
8. Have you attended a stress-management, relaxation, time-management or assertiveness-training course? ❏
9. Do you show Type B behavior (*see* p. 22)? ❏

PART 2

10. Do you smoke? ❏
11. Do you drink alcohol to relax? ❏
12. Do you take sleeping pills? ❏
13. Do you take work home? ❏
14. Do you drink more than eight cups of caffeinated drinks (coffee, tea, cola, hot chocolate) a day? ❏
15. Do you show Type A behavior (*see* pp. 16–22)? ❏

How did you score?

PART 1

Q1. Yes, 20 points
Q2. Yes, 10 points
Q3. Yes, 5 points; 10 if you go more than once a month
Q4. Yes, 15 points

Q5. Yes, 10 points

Q6. Yes, 20 points

Q7. Yes, 10 points

Q8. Yes, 10 points for each course you attend

Q9. Yes, 15 points

Add up your score for good coping strategies. ☐

PART 2

Q10. Yes, minus 10 points for every 20 cigarettes you smoke each day.

Q11. Yes, minus 10 points for every 10 servings of alcohol drunk each week above recommended limits (which are 14 servings for women and 21 servings for men, where a serving is a 5 oz. glass of wine, half a pint of beer or one ounce of spirits).

Q12. Yes, minus 10 points

Q13. Yes, minus 5 points for each night of the week that you take work home

Q14. Yes, minus 5 points for every 5 cups over 8 cups per day

Q15. Yes, check your Type A behavior assessment (see pp. 18–20): minus 5 points if you scored between 40 and 60; 10 points if you scored between 60 and 70; and 15 if you score more than 70.

Add up your score for poor coping strategies. ☐

For your overall coping ability score, subtract your part 2 score from part 1 score.

What does your score mean? A positive score means that you have good coping ability. The higher the score the better able you are to deal with the pressures and demands that you face.

A negative score indicates that you have poor coping ability. The lower your score, the lower your ability to deal with the pressures and demands that you face and the greater your need to develop strategies for dealing with stress in your life.

Stress-related Ailments

Long-term stress, where the fight or flight response is continually switched on without sufficient time to relax between spurts of work, can lead to chronic exhaustion and illness. Research has found that people who go through a stressful life crisis, such as bereavement, marital breakdown or moving to a new house, may show a significant impairment in their body's immune system.

When our body is under constant stress it keeps on producing increased amounts of stress hormones, particularly cortisol (*see* p. 9). This hormone has a depressing effect on the immune system. Tests on people experiencing high levels of stress have found a reduction in the activity of the body's natural killer cells which are an essential part of the immune system. These cells roam around the blood system on the lookout for and ready to attack foreign bodies and destroy any mutant cancer cells. Research has shown that relaxation boosts the activity of the killer cells and so helps to strengthen the immune system.

The following are all common illnesses in which stress can play a part.

ALLERGIES

An oversensitivity to certain foods, plants, animals or insect bites which can cause eczema, migraines, rashes, fatigue, nausea, sneezing, wheezing and diarrhea.

Allergies occur when our body's immune system treats substances such as pollen or peanuts as if they are dangerous invaders. Inhaling or coming into contact with even tiny amounts of the offending substance or allergen, as it is known, will trigger the immune system to release substances called antibodies. Chemicals called histamines are then released causing the inflammation and irritated skin and membranes commonly associated with allergies. It is often the case that when a person is stressed, and their body is working overtime, they suddenly find that they suffer an allergic reaction to foods or substances that never affected them in the past.

COMMON ALLERGENS INCLUDE:

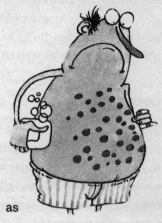

- animal hair
- feathers
- pollen
- detergents/soap
- cosmetics
- milk
- cheese
- wheat flour
- shellfish
- nuts
- chocolate
- food additives, such as artificial colorings

CANCER

Research shows that the way in which we deal with stress can affect the progression of some cancers, and a number of studies have focused on the connection between our emotions, hormones and physical reaction.

Studies have shown that women with a positive mental attitude towards breast cancer had a greater chance of recovery than women whose attitudes were negative. It is important to be able to discuss your feelings rather than bottling them up. A study of skin cancer patients showed that those who refused to admit to feeling afraid or angry had the most rapidly advancing cancers.

If someone close to you is diagnosed as having cancer, encourage them to talk about their feelings about the disease as well as their physical symptoms.

COLDS

The Common Cold Research Unit investigated the effect of stress on susceptibility to colds, and found that anxiety had a pronounced effect on the participants involved in the study. It has also been found that seemingly unrelated illnesses, including viral infections, seem to come in clusters after periods of stress.

DEPRESSION

Long-term stress, combined with other factors such as personality, environment, genes and upbringing can lead to full-blown depression (as opposed to the normal feeling of being a bit down that we all experience from time to time).

Stress and depression have many symptoms in common. If you experience four or more of the symptoms listed on the following page and have done so for more than two weeks, in spite of your attempts to shake them off, it would be advisable to consult your doctor:

- loss of interest and enjoyment in life
- lack of motivation, so that even simple tasks and decisions are impossible
- complete fatigue
- significant loss or gain in appetite or weight
- sleeplessness or excessive sleeping
- no interest in physical affection or sex
- loss of self-confidence and avoiding meeting people
- irritability
- feeling useless, inadequate, bad, helpless and hopeless
- feeling worse at certain times of day, usually the morning
- thoughts of suicide

DIABETES

Physical or emotional stress is unlikely to cause diabetes in a healthy person. But if you are inactive, overweight and smoke, stress may trigger the onset of adult-onset or non-insulin-dependent (Type 2) diabetes. This condition is less severe but more common than insulin-dependent (Type 1) diabetes. It tends to develop slowly over years, often without symptoms, and as a result, it frequently goes undiagnosed.

FERTILITY

High levels of stress have been found to lower fertility due to the hormone changes that take place in the body. This can also contribute to menstrual problems, such as very heavy, painful periods.

HAIR LOSS

Stress can result in alopecia areata in which hair falls out by the handful, leaving unsightly bald patches. It can affect the scalp, eyebrows and body hair. Once the period of stress is over, the hair usually grows back.

HEADACHES

Stress is a well-recognized cause of tension and migraine headaches. Muscles that are tense from hours of concentration, sitting hunched over a desk or in an awkward position, or from hours spent in difficult meetings or driving, will often set off a headache.

A migraine headache comes on as a result of the spasms and relaxation of the blood vessels covering the brain and symptoms can include nausea, vomiting and sensitivity to light. Migraine sufferers should keep a diary to help them identify the factors that seem to cause headaches.

HEART DISEASE

Stressful emotions such as anxiety, fear and hostility can trigger the release of stress hormones into the bloodstream, put the heart into overdrive and cause angina attacks. If the blood supply to the heart is restricted by clogged arteries and the person's life is also very stressful, a heart attack may result. Anyone who suffers from heart problems must take urgent steps to reduce the stress in their lives.

HIGH BLOOD PRESSURE

Our blood pressure rises and falls numerous times a day whenever we exert ourselves or our emotions are aroused. It also rises in response to stressful situations. In general it will return to normal once the period of stress is over.

Sometimes, however, if the rise is severe or prolonged, changes occur in the arteries which cause the blood pressure to stay high. High blood pressure tends to run in families, so it makes even more sense to learn how to deal with stress if you think you might have a genetic predisposition to the condition.

IRRITABLE BOWEL SYNDROME

Frequent abdominal pains and cramps, bloating, diarrhea, constipation, and even heartburn (though less often), can be signs of irritable bowel syndrome (IBS).

Many sufferers of IBS can trace the start of their symptoms to a stressful event such as exams, marital problems, financial difficulties or bereavement. Young adults tend to develop IBS because they find their lives generally stressful. Research has shown that anxiety can lead to an overactive bowel.

When stress levels are high the bowels of IBS sufferers contract more than those of non-sufferers. The resulting spasm is what causes the pain, which in turn produces more stress, creating a vicious circle of stress, spasm and pain. There are a number of treatments to alleviate the symptoms of IBS but none will be effective long-term if the cause is not addressed.

PANIC ATTACKS

Long-term anxiety can lead to feelings of panic which seem to come out of the blue and which can be frightening and debilitating. Some techniques for coping with panic attacks are described on pp. 175–79.

PEPTIC ULCERS

Many experts now believe that peptic ulcers are caused by a type of bacteria called H pylori and not stress, as was the commonly held view for many years. However there is no question that stress can worsen the condition by increasing the level of gastric acid in the stomach.

SKIN DISEASES

Conditions such as eczema, urticaria (hives), acne and psoriasis are all worsened by stress and in some cases are directly caused by it. Often the unsightliness of these conditions can cause embarrassment to sufferers which in turn induces further stress and a vicious cycle results.

TAKE ACTION

If you suffer from any of the ailments listed, it is vital that you address the causes of stress in your life as well as seeking medical help for the physical symptoms. It may be that you have to leave a job that is putting you under too much pressure, sell a house with an expensive mortgage and move somewhere cheaper, or seek counseling to help you deal with relationships that are causing you grief. Check the **A–Z of Stressful Situations** for advice on dealing with the specific events that cause you stress.

AN A-Z OF
STRESSFUL
SITUATIONS

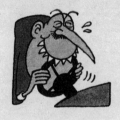

Accidents

How much attention do you pay to breaking a glass or stubbing your toe on a table leg? These are accidents that happen every day of the week. You clear up the glass, or hop around until the pain in your toe subsides and then carry on with life.

However, a more serious accident, such as a car crash, will be much harder to come to terms with, not only because its scale is so much greater, but because serious accidents often undermine our basic belief system. Very serious accidents are also referred to as trauma. After a person has been through a shocking or life-threatening experience, he or she may go on to develop debilitating psychological or physiological symptoms collectively called post-traumatic stress disorder (PTSD). Research has shown that a single terrifying event can alter the brain chemistry and trigger further adrenaline surges which result in panic attacks, anxiety, confusion, dreams, intrusive thoughts and flashbacks.

PTSD is common among soldiers readjusting to life at the end of a war, but is not limited to them. Survivors of earthquakes, fires, train and plane crashes, people who have been involved in or witnessed a murder, can also experience PTSD. However, you don't have to be directly involved in an event to experience trauma. Very often relatives and friends of victims and even rescue workers will be left feeling traumatized by an event. Whether or not a person goes on to develop PTSD depends partially on the support he or she receives from others and on how willing they are to accept help.

STRESSBUSTERS

- Try to get back to normal life as soon as possible.
- Don't bottle up your emotions; accept that you may feel numb for a time. Talk through the incident with friends and play it back in your mind. Don't go out of the way to avoid triggers that may bring back painful memories.
- Look after yourself: eat well, build in relaxation time and get plenty of sleep. Put aside some time to be alone or just with family and close friends.
- Accidents are more common after a stressful event so be extra vigilant around the home and when driving.

- With time, most people overcome PTSD, but if your symptoms persist beyond a few months you should seek professional help. Counseling or psychotherapy are often effective. Cognitive and behavioral therapy where the patient relives the traumatic event have helped PTSD symptoms in rape victims.

Bosses

There are three main relationships in the work-place: with our colleagues, with those junior to us, and with our superiors. The last of these is arguably one of the greatest causes of stress at work.

Working with a boss whom we respect and trust can make time spent in the office or on the factory floor a highly productive and satisfying time. But a difficult boss can make the nine-to-five a living hell. In general, difficult bosses can be put into one of two groups: the bad boss or the bully.

SIX SIGNS OF A BAD BOSS

Here's how to spot if your boss is the cause of your stress at work. He/she:

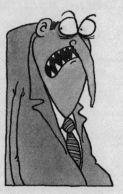

- can't or won't delegate
- spends the day in meetings
- picks favorites and plays staff off against each other

- expects you to put work before your personal life
- never gives praise for a job well done but always lets everyone know when you have made a mistake
- never listens to employees' or customers' complaints

COULD YOUR BOSS BE A BULLY?

The bullying boss is a growing phenomenon. One reason is because in this day and age jobs are increasingly less secure, thus making people more vulnerable to their managers. Two out of every three middle managers believe that bullying is a major cause of workplace stress, according to a 1997 survey.

There are two kinds of bully. Most common is the boss who is also under a huge amount of stress and pressure. He or she can't cope and so takes it out on those junior to him- or herself.

Then there's the bully who has always been a bully: vicious and vindictive in private, he or she is all smiles and charm when others are around. If you answer yes to six or more of the following questions, chances are that you are being picked on and are well within you rights to complain.

- Does the working relationship between you and your boss feel different from any you have experienced with previous bosses?
- Do you constantly feel "picked on"?
- Is your work criticized even though it is of a high standard?
- Is your boss new?
- Is your boss under growing pressure?
- Are your workload/objectives constantly changed?
- Are you frequently asked to perform tasks outside your job description?
- Are you being put under increased personal scrutiny?
- Do you feel increasingly less involved?

See also **Colleagues, Work.**

STRESSBUSTERS

- Ask for feedback from your boss, and be prepared for a frank comment.
- Try not to take every critical comment to heart or let others' judgment sway you unduly.
- If you feel your boss is holding you back consider changing your job.
- Be relaxed and positive with your boss. Smile and greet them by name. Inquire about their personal life.

- Assert yourself, stand your ground and look your boss in the eye.
- If your boss is a bully:

  - avoid the temptation to lash out. He/she may fight back and the situation can quickly escalate into a fist-fight, and you may find yourself bullied more, sacked on the spot or arrested for assault.
  - write down any incidents that occur, no matter how trivial: what was said and when, your response and how you felt. Speak to anyone who could have seen or heard what happened. If things get very bad, your lawyer will need this evidence.
  - talk to your family and friends about what's going on.
  - find out if any of your colleagues are being bullied, then report it to your personnel director or your boss's boss and tell them what is going on. This way your claim will seem like less of a personality clash problem. Make sure that you see someone in a very senior position within the organization so that something can be done.
  - make your complaint official. Check your contract or company handbook for your terms and conditions of employment to see if your com-

pany has an official grievance procedure, and use it to lodge your complaint. In a small company where the bully may also be the owner, be prepared to look outside the company for help.

Cars

*"Our motor car is our supreme form of privacy
when away from home."*

Marshall McLuhan

When you jump into your car and turn on the ignition, does it fire into action, or does it splutter and scream before finally turning over? Nothing is more frustrating than a car that won't start when you are desperate to get somewhere. Whether you are driving the latest Jaguar off the production line or an old jalopy you should ask yourself, is your car your lifeline or a weight around your neck?

If you can only afford an old car that develops frequent problems, you will need to have a good understanding of mechanics to keep it on the road, and even new cars can have problems. Cars can be a massive drain on your finances, when you add up the cost of gas, tolls, insurance, parking, tires and general maintenance. And because cars are not cheap, you will be concerned to protect yours and upset by the slightest scratch or the tiniest patch of rust that appears.

Cars are still too often regarded by men as a man's world. Women can be patronized and treated as stupid by garage mechanics and car dealers. Prepare by reading a couple of magazines before you walk in to a car showroom and buy a service or repair manual for your car.

See also **Driving, Road Rage.**

STRESSBUSTERS

- Have your car regularly checked and serviced.
- Keep tires at the correct pressure—check them once every two weeks and before going on long journeys.
- Find a reliable garage or mechanic who can explain problems and the expenses that might be involved. Ask your friends for recommendations.
- If you are unfortunate enough to develop a serious problem, get a couple of quotes from different sources before deciding who you want to do the work.

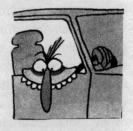

- Attend a short car maintenance course that explains the basic tasks you must do regularly to avoid bigger problems. This should include checking the oil, water, tire pressure, changing light bulbs, and so on.

• Join AAA or another roadside assistance service. The expense is worth the peace of mind.

• Every now and then, consider whether you really need to have a car or if you could manage better (and more cheaply) by using public transportation and taxis.

Changing Careers

"If what you are doing is making you sick then stop doing it."

Abraham Maslow

What happens when you are fed up with your career in advertising sales and want to give it all up to become a landscape gardener? Do you decide that you are too old to jump ship and stay put, or do you pay attention to what your inner voice is telling you and act on it?

Change is never easy. But if your job constantly puts you in a rotten mood, it could be hazardous to your health. Research has found that women in highly stressful jobs with a low level of control are likely to be depressed, anxious and hostile—factors that are known to boost the risk of heart disease and undermine the immune system.

In some careers people naturally move into new roles as they age: professional athletes often become coaches. But not everyone makes such an obvious transition—actors becoming politicians is a less obvious but not unprecedented example.

There are a few careers that you may be too old for—prima ballerinas and world-class athletes rarely start in their 40s—and sometimes it's hard to figure out how you could support yourself during retraining. But try to think positively and find solutions to the problems rather than giving up at the first fence. It could be well worth it.

STRESSBUSTERS

- Talk to your family/friends and enlist their support.
- It is easier to find a new job if you are already employed.
- Test the water before jumping ship.
- Talk to your bank about a career development loan. The interest charged is lower than for normal loans and you don't have to start paying it back till six months after your training is completed.
- Find out as much as you can about your new career to make sure you have the necessary experience. Do you need to retrain or can you learn on the job?

- Speak to people in the business or consult a career adviser.
- Talk to people who have already changed careers—they may be able to give you invaluable advice, as well as being living proof that a career change is achievable.
- Practice positive affirmations to help keep you focused on your goal (*see* page 223).

Children

"Never have children, only grandchildren."
Gore Vidal, Two Sisters

Bringing up children is mainly guesswork, and in today's busy world the relationship between parents and their children is often a highly charged one. Arguments about the time spent with children and striking the right balance between home life and work pressures is a problem common to many families. Not to mention the worry that all parents face over their children's health, education and responsibility for their future. And it's not just parents who have the worries; it's very stressful being a child in our competitive, modern society.

The feeling that as a parent you "may not be doing the right thing" can create a certain amount of stress. But there is no "absolute" right or wrong way to raise kids.

Clinical research has found that the most important things that you can do for your children are to ensure that they grow up feeling loved for who they are not what they do, and to help them to communicate and express the whole range of human emotions.

STRESSBUSTERS

- Be honest, open and direct with your children.
- Find time to have fun together.
- Help them to understand that all feelings and emotions are natural, but that they will have to learn self-control when appropriate.
- Be authoritative, but also listen to their views and discuss issues with them.
- Do not expect your children to follow suit as the next in a long line of doctors, for example—respect them and encourage them to develop and pursue their own interests.
- Share parental power and swap roles to avoid one parent always being responsible for discipline. If you are a single parent, try to find another adult (a grandparent or friend) who can help to share the burden and listen when you need to discuss worries about the children.
- Watch out for changes in your child's behavior,

such as loss of appetite, withdrawal or lack of interest. These may indicate a deeper problem, such as bullying.

As a parent it's important to try to understand your children—what they like and dislike, what they're afraid of—and remember that as your children get older the problems they experience multiply. By the time they are adolescents they face increasing pressure to start thinking about their future careers and go on to higher education. One of the ways in which this pressure manifests itself in today's society is through drug and alcohol abuse. In the U.S. and Japan youth suicides are the leading cause of death among teenagers. The main sources of stress among adolescents are their attempts to meet the often conflicting expectations of parents, teachers and peer groups.

STEPCHILDREN

Taking on stepchildren is highly stressful for both step- and biological-parents, who may feel guilty for not really loving their new child or for disrupting their child's life, while children may feel angry with step-parents for trying to replace their natural parent. Add to that the jealousy and rivalry between siblings from different marriages, and it's little wonder that relationships in step-families are even more highly charged than in natural families.

- Discuss with your stepchild the kind of relationship you both feel you should have. You may get along better as friends than as parent and child.
- Don't criticize their biological parent in front of the child.
- Try to take an interest in your stepchild's biological family so that they don't feel they have a separate life which they cannot discuss with you.

Colleagues

"Good relationships between members of a group are a key factor in individual and organizational health."

Dr. Hans Selye, stress researcher

We spend around a third of our lives at work, so the relationships we have with our colleagues—good or bad—will have a big impact on our lives. Our colleagues should be a source of support, friendship and camaraderie, which can help us to cope with stressful situations. Supportive colleagues will encourage and help a co-worker while they are resolving a difficult problem.

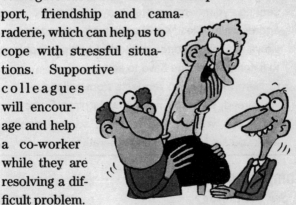

But work relationships can also be a huge source of stress, particularly if there is an atmosphere of competition or if there are personality clashes in the workplace.

STRESSBUSTERS

For your relationship with colleagues to thrive, you need:

- to give and receive support.
- good communication skills (knowing when to assert yourself and when to compromise is a skill that can be learned).
- the ability to listen—not only will you learn more about people by listening, but you will also develop better relationships.
- to avoid raising your voice in discussion and presenting your arguments too emotionally or aggressively. Clearly and assertively stating your views is a much better method of getting people to listen to what you have to say.
- to learn to say no to requests from colleagues if you already have too much on your plate. Be honest about why you are refusing, so they don't think you are just being uncooperative.

Computers
See **Technology**

Cooking

"Men cook to show off, women cook to please."

With the number of cookery programs, magazines and column space in newspapers devoted to preparing food, you'd think that everyone loved cooking. But for those who face the task of preparing family meals seven days a week, time spent in the kitchen is not as rosy as the Reynolds Wrap ads would have us believe.

In most cases this job falls to the woman of the house, who often has a job to hold down too. Hand-in-hand with the task of cooking comes the weekly

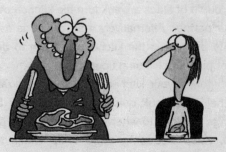

shopping trip to the supermarket—a stress-packed event in itself (*see* **Shopping**).

And that's just the start: there's also the fact that your eldest child has decided to become a vegetarian. Which would be no trouble except for the fact that your husband doesn't consider he's eaten a proper meal if there's no meat on his plate. And so it goes on.

STRESSBUSTERS

- Before the weekly shopping trip get everyone to say what they would like to eat in the following week and write out the week's shopping list based on their suggestions. Failure to give full answers means they have to eat what they are given with no complaints.
- Know what you are going to cook and stick to it. Changing your mind several times can be exhausting.
- Get your children involved in helping to prepare the meal as soon as they are old enough.
- A couple of times a week turn the kitchen over to your partner. Alternatively if he or she is a complete disaster in the kitchen get them to do the shopping and clearing up instead.
- Reorganize your kitchen. Is everything arranged to help you cook quickly and efficiently? Store things as close to where they are used as possible. Keep frequently used tools within arm's

reach. Clear away from worktops everything that is not often used.

- Have a couple of ready-prepared meals in the freezer for those times you can't be bothered to cook from scratch.
- Treat yourself to take-out now and again.

Crime

"The fear of burglars is not only the fear of being robbed, but also the fear of a sudden and unexpected clutch out of the darkness."
Elias Canetti, Crowds and Power

In today's increasingly violent world, tales of horrific crimes are becoming more and more common. For some victims of violent assault—physical or emotional—the feelings of distress are so profound that they lead to post-traumatic stress disorder (PTSD). For more information on this, *see* **Accidents**.

The most severe cases occur when the threat to the victim's safety is overwhelming and their sense of personal control is lost. Not all victims of crime will develop PTSD, but those who try to downplay the extent to which they have been affected or who refuse to talk about it may be at greater risk. Rape victims, for example, who are criticized by their spouse or partner are more likely to develop PTSD than those who feel supported.

The effects of a crime can be suffered years after the event and can sometimes get out of control. It is natural to feel nervous about walking home after dark when you have been a crime victim, but once it starts to prevent you leading a full life because you're turning down invitations to events you used to enjoy, then it is time to seek help. You may decide to install an alarm system after a burglary but if your home has become like Fort Knox with panic buttons all over the place, this will serve as a constant reminder of what happened rather than be a source of security.

For some people, fear of crime can become as debilitating as the event itself. Take proper precautions to ensure your safety and then relax and remember that, statistically, you are very unlikely to become a target of any serious crime.

STRESSBUSTERS

- Don't think that you have to cope on your own. Help is available from a variety of sources.
- If you are the victim of domestic violence, dial 911 in an emergency. At other times contact the Domestic Violence Unit at your local police station. The staff there are specially trained to deal with your situation.
- Specially trained police officers are available to offer counseling to victims of rape and other harrowing experiences.

- If you are on the receiving end of malicious telephone calls, don't reveal any details about yourself, put down the handset immediately and try to stay calm. Report any such calls to the police and, if the calls continue, consider changing your phone number.

Death

*"Guilt is perhaps the most painful companion
of death."*

Elisabeth Kübler-Ross

The death of a loved one is regarded as one of the most stressful life events you can face. Whether your loss is sudden or expected it leaves the mind and body feeling empty. Coming to terms with and learning to adjust to personal loss is a painful and stressful process.

Many people feel a sense of guilt, that they weren't perhaps the ideal husband, wife, daughter or son. There may have been an argument with the deceased person that had not been resolved. It is important that you talk these feelings through with a close friend or a counselor and don't allow them to get out of control.

Four recognized stages of grief have been identified—though not everyone will go through all four.

1. **Shock:** this is a period of denial and disbelief, hysteria and confusion. These emotions all help to protect you by slowing down the speed at which reality sinks in.
2. **Protest:** this stage is characterized by powerful feelings of anger, guilt, sadness, fear, yearning and searching.
3. **Disorganization:** reality has sunk in and the loss becomes very real. Feelings of bleakness, despair, apathy, anxiety and confusion are commonly experienced in this stage.
4. **Reorganization:** you start to put your life back together and feel strong enough to look to happier times. At this stage people often find that their basic values have changed and may even discover a new meaning in life.

As with any trauma or shock, you need to give yourself time to grieve. Just how much time differs from person to person, and can take years.

STRESSBUSTERS

- Take one day at a time. With time you will begin to feel better. One of the worst things you can do is to believe that you have to cope with everything and everyone immediately.
- Talk honestly about how you feel. This includes expressing any regrets that you may have. Talk

about your fears, your loneliness, anger or sadness. You don't have to "behave well" or put on a brave face.

- Look after yourself. During stressful times it is vital that you act, work and care for yourself as you would for a close friend.
- Speak to a professional. Enlisting the help of a trained counselor to work through your loss with you can be very helpful. A counselor will provide a safe environment and a framework in which you can express and confront your feelings.

Discrimination

Discrimination comes in many forms. Where once discrimination took place or was only recognized as taking place along racial or ethnic lines, today it is a very different picture. Gender, sexual orientation, race, disability and age are all areas in which any of us can find ourselves the victims of discrimination.

Being the target of discrimination is incredibly distressing, mainly because people are unsure as to the course of action they should take. Remember that discrimination is against the law, and stand up for your rights.

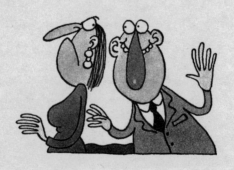

STRESSBUSTERS

- For workplace discrimination of any type, speak to your line manager, personnel director or union.
- For racial discrimination outside the workplace, call the police or one of the many organizations set up to combat this offense.
- For discrimination at school, speak to your family and principal.

Divorce

Going through a divorce is thought to be the second most stressful life event after the death of a partner or spouse. Whether the separation is amicable or messy, divorce and the prospect of facing life alone is hard on both sexes. And there is no easy way through it. The emotional turmoil experienced is often likened to mourning. Feelings of disbelief, anger, sadness and the loss of emotional support, all have to be worked through before you can move on.

Your circle of friends and acquaintances will most probably have shrunk as at least some of your mutual friends will inevitably take sides. Having to deal with household tasks that your partner may once have done can cause feelings of resentment, self-pity and inadequacy. And if you have children or financial worries or both, this will only add to your sense of exhaustion and stress.

To a certain extent, marriage and all that it entails—happiness, mental health, career success—benefits men more than women. So men, contrary to appearances, tend to have more to lose in a divorce than women. Women are more often given custody of children and limited contact with their children can be a source of suffering for men that is not always acknowledged by society in general. More men suffer mental health problems after a divorce, reporting symptoms such as despair, helplessness, mood swings, withdrawal and suicidal thoughts.

Try to give yourself time and resist the urge to contemplate the distant future until your divorce is at least a year old.

STRESSBUSTERS

- Make contact with people in the same boat; join a divorced or single-parent group.
- Ask for help from your friends and family. Confide in others and don't be afraid to cry—it will help to relieve stress and pain.
- Remind yourself that the pain you are experiencing is a process you will come through.
- Fill your time. Get out of the house every day through work, hobbies, charity work and leisure.

- Don't pry into your ex-partner's new life.
- Look after yourself; don't let your appearance slip.
- Make your home as relaxing and as comfortable as possible; redecorate, listen to music and make yourself nutritious meals.

Drinking

"Even though a number of people have tried, no one has yet found a way to drink for a living."
Jean Kerr, Poor Richard

Having a couple of drinks at the end of a stressful day is a way to wind down and relax. But when even a minor crisis has you reaching for a bottle of wine you should look carefully at your dependency on alcohol.

In heavily stressful times it is common to turn to alcohol for solace or to lift our spirits. However, the benefits of this kind of approach are strictly short-term. Drinking heavily on a regular basis will not help you to deal with the root of your stress and can lead to long-term problems. Remember too, that while social drinking can help to enliven your mood, if you are drinking because you feel stressed or angry, drinking can have the opposite effect. In addition, many people report that they feel more anxious and less able to cope the day after a drinking binge.

Alcohol is a depressant and not a stimulant; it will dull your memory and concentration, making 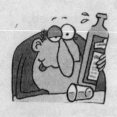 it difficult to cope with the demands of everyday life. Excessive drinking can damage your brain, liver, digestive tract and stomach. It disrupts your sleep patterns, and puts a strain on relationships.

Drinking can set off mood swings and erratic or irresponsible behavior that can put your partner and children under stress. So turning to alcohol to help you deal with stress will just exacerbate the problem.

STRESSBUSTERS

- Be clear in your own mind as to why you are drinking. Do you drink because:

  - you are bored
  - it helps you to relax
  - it gives you confidence
  - you are under pressure
  - you feel you need it in social situations
  - you feel lonely
  - you are depressed

- Decide beforehand what your limit will be for the evening and stick to it. Don't let others pressurize you into drinking more.

- Alternate alcoholic drinks with soft drinks.
- Vary when and where you drink.
- Try not to drink every day.
- Don't drink when you feel lonely, depressed, stressed or need confidence, or to make you more outgoing.

Driving

When you get behind the wheel of your car, are you a demon who burns rubber or do you consider and respect the other drivers on the road? Driving like a bat out of hell may make you feel as if you are covering a lot of ground, but in a busy metropoli-

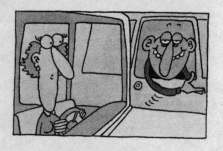

tan area this approach won't get you very far, and will only send your stress levels soaring. Having said that, driving over-cautiously does not necessarily make you a safer driver: it can give the impression of uncertainty and a lack of confidence and road sense. This can be just as hazardous for other drivers as being a road hog.

STRESSBUSTERS

- Drive with due care and diligence, keep within the law and respect the other drivers on the road.
- Take regular breaks on long journeys.
- Don't drive if you are overtired.
- Build in time for delays.

Drugs

At times of great emotional stress we often turn to drugs to help us sleep or to calm us down. As well as the more socially acceptable drugs such as alcohol and nicotine, medical drugs such as tranquilizers and sleeping pills and so-called "recreational" drugs such as marijuana and cocaine are used for their mood- or mind-altering properties.

It is not totally clear how these drugs affect the brain or why some people become physically dependent on them. However two clear signs of a physical dependence or addiction are:

- taking greater doses to achieve the same effect
- painful withdrawal symptoms

Some drugs will cause one or the other of the above, while heroin, for example, will cause both. Smoking marijuana does not lead to a true physical dependence but it can create a psychological one.

In the short term, prescription drugs such as tranquilizers or sleeping pills can be a useful aid in coping with stress. In the long term, however, they only mask the symptoms and do not deal with the cause of the anxiety. At the same time they can lower self-confidence and cause a range of physical side-effects including drowsiness, dry mouth, dizziness, change in appetite and poor coordination, any of which can impair your ability to carry out everyday tasks.

While not all users will become dependent on drugs, there are real risks associated with taking any drug. For some, these risks can be very serious.

If you suspect that your child might be taking drugs, watch out for the following signs:

- unusual moods, restlessness and irritability
- excessive spending or borrowing of money
- sores or rashes around the mouth
- poor appetite
- dilated or constricted pupils

Drug paraphernalia can include metal tins, pill boxes, plastic, cellophane or foil wrappers, twists of paper, sugar cubes, used matches, shredded cigarettes, and torn pieces of paper. If you find something suspicious, ask your child about it in a low-key way.

STRESSBUSTERS

- If you believe that you may be dependent on drugs talk to your doctor about the problem. He or she may not treat you but will be able to provide you with information about local drug clinics where help is available and, if necessary, refer you for psychiatric help.

Eating Disorders

Eating disorders can be roughly split into two groups: anorexia nervosa and bulimia nervosa. Both conditions most frequently affect females from middle-class backgrounds, aged between 10 and 40 years old. However, eating disorders are becoming more common among males.

Anorexia and bulimia nervosa arise from deep-rooted anxiety. Other predisposing factors include low self-esteem, perfectionism, feelings of powerlessness and cultural/social pressure to be slim. Anorexics starve themselves and are usually very thin. In severe cases sufferers may be hospitalized to prevent them from starving to death.

Bulimics binge on fattening foods then purge by making themselves vomit or by taking laxatives. Bulimia is often hard to detect. Weight is not an immediate indicator as sufferers can be normal weight or even overweight. And they will try to conceal their behavior.

Signs of bulimia include:

- going to the toilet after every meal
- mood swings
- secretive behavior
- the use of a large amount of laxatives
- in the long-term bulimics' tooth enamel can be eroded because vomiting has bathed their teeth in stomach acids and their intestines can be seriously damaged

The dividing line between anorexia and bulimia is blurred by the fact that 50 percent of all anorexics binge and purge even at very low weights. Bulimics sometimes switch between periods of strict dieting and binging. It is also fairly common for anorexics to become bulimic.

STRESSBUSTERS

- Be honest with yourself.
- Discuss your feelings frankly with your doctor and/ or psychotherapist and with your family, if you can.
- Take a good multivitamin and mineral supplement. Both anorexics and bulimics tend to be deficient in magnesium, vitamin B1, zinc and potassium.
- Learn to recognize the situations which trigger a binge and develop strategies for dealing with them.
- Parents who suspect their child may have an eating disorder should seek professional help.

Exams and Tests

"Interviews, exams and tests are easy; the fears, the doubts and the uncertainties that surround these events often are not."

Robert Holden

When it comes to your driving test, school exams, university degrees, job interviews, professional qualifications, auditions, social club entrance interviews or work presentations, it's the fear of failure, the nervous anticipation and the self-doubt rather than the test itself that is stressful.

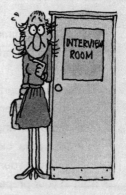

Fear of failure can lead to two reactions: self-doubt, or the will to succeed. The trick is to use your nervous energy to motivate yourself rather than let it eat away at your self-confidence and self-esteem. The other key strategy is to prepare—develop a plan that will enable you to learn all you need to know and keep your stress levels in check.

Some people can actually become physically ill before exams or job interviews, and they may need professional advice to overcome their problems. This could involve some form of counseling to look at why they feel quite so pressurized—perhaps they are trying to live up to impossible ideals set by parents, teachers or siblings. Hypnotherapists can also teach some useful techniques for calming severe cases of pre-exam nerves (see pp. 195–96). And read **Quick tips for beating stress** on pp. 175–85.

STRESSBUSTERS

- Plan the time leading up to your exam, interview or test.
- Commit yourself to doing your best.
- Plan a revision timetable.
- Identify and work on your weak spots.
- Practice your performance— look at old exam papers, take more driving lessons as your test gets closer, present a sales plan to colleagues or your boss.
- Trust in your preparation to see you through.

Flying

"I feel about airplanes the way I feel about diets. It seems to me that they are wonderful things for other people to go on."
Jean Kerr, The Snake Has All the Lines

Flying is said to be 25 times safer than driving, yet aerophobia—fear of flying—affects thousands of people. So much so that the very thought of boarding a plane brings out a cold sweat or induces a panic attack. Some resort to tranquilizers before flying while others sedate themselves with alcohol in the departure lounge (but note that the airline will not let you on board if you are obviously intoxicated).

Airlines such as British Airways offer a one-day confidence-boosting course, aimed at helping nervous fliers to understand and control their fear. On the course aerophobics learn about flying and practice relaxation techniques before ending the day with a short flight.

For some people, understanding the science of

how airplanes fly helps. The principles of aerodynamics are such that it takes something very major and extraordinary to go wrong to cause a crash.

See the coping strategies listed below, try to master some relaxation techniques (*see* pp. 197–209) and consider some of the therapies suggested for dealing with **Phobias**, such as counselling and hypnotherapy.

STRESSBUSTERS

To overcome your aerophobia try the following program:

- At least four months before your flight begin relaxation training.
- In a state of relaxation, visualize the airport and the plane. Picture yourself feeling calm and confident.
- Try to visit the airport before you fly; sit in the lounge and relax.
- On the day of your flight practice relaxation techniques while you wait to board your plane. While in the air, focus all your attention on relaxing. Breathe calmly and slowly, imagining that you are at home sitting in your favorite armchair. Concentrate on your breathing and relax your hands.

Formal Occasions

Weddings, christenings and funerals are emotion-ally charged occasions, whether you are arrang-ing or just attending them. As with any big gathering a certain amount of stress will be involved. But when the majority of those attending are family members the stress quotient is far higher. If you are in charge of the organization, the key to keeping your stress levels to a minimum is deciding on the kind of occasion you want, setting a budget and sticking to it.

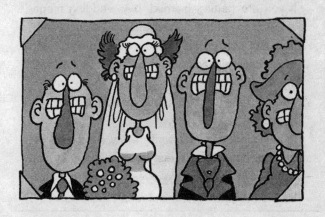

On the day itself, the pressure for everything to be perfect is immense but you must resist it. The chances are that something will go wrong but remember that these incidents are not important in the long term. It is the sentiments behind the occasion that count.

STRESSBUSTERS

- If you are going to be in charge of organizing a funeral for a relative or friend who has been ill for some time, talk to them about the kind of service they would want. If that is too difficult, ask them to write their wishes in their will.
- Delegate—don't do everything yourself.
- If you are planning a fairly large event, hire outside caterers to help.
- Prepare as much as you can in advance.
- If you are getting married, buy wedding magazines or one of the many useful books on the subject. Not only do they usually contain some kind of wedding planner, but they are also stuffed with information on everything from where to rent classic cars or hire tents to tips on making speeches.
- If guests are coming from far away, send out a list of local hotels and guest houses—that way you won't have the additional stress of putting people up in your home.

- Keep lists of things to do as the event gets closer. Review your list each day to ensure that nothing gets missed.

Friends

Who do you turn to in stressful times? Your family, your partner, a good friend or all three? The chances are it's probably your oldest friend.

Friends can be a source of stress. But they can also be a great support during stressful times. Research has shown that women with at least one good friend in whom they could confide were 90 percent less likely to become depressed than those women without close friends. It is the quality of friends, not the quantity that's important here. And a good friend should be treasured like a priceless jewel.

STRESSBUSTERS

To maintain a stress-free friendship:

- Let them win an argument occasionally; be the first to apologize.
- Don't say anything behind their back that you wouldn't say to their face.
- Listen.
- Be prepared to share in a friend's failure.
- Accept them for who they are—warts and all.

Guests

"The first day a man is a guest, the second a burden, the third a pest."

Edouard Laboulaye

Having friends to stay can be an eagerly antici-
pated event that turns into a nightmare. As the
host, no matter how welcome your visitors are, you
will be aware that your personal daily routine will be
affected, and time to yourself will be almost non-

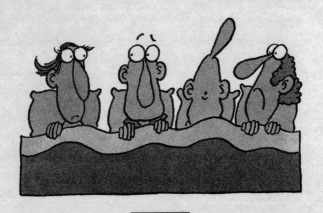

existent. You will also tend to look after everyone except yourself.

As the guest, being away from home and living out of a suitcase can be very unsettling no matter how comfortable you are made to feel. And unless the house is large, the lack of physical space will be felt by everyone.

STRESSBUSTERS

- Plan plenty of activities.
- Don't feel that you have to accompany your guests on every outing—it will give you and them some time and space. Use that time to relax—have a long bath or a nap.
- Share responsibilities. As the host don't feel that you have to do all the chores. Equally as the guest don't assume that you have to be waited on around the clock. Help with chores, offer to cook a meal.
- Both parties should put some money aside, so that they can enjoy the visit properly.

Before any visit, it will help if the ground rules are firmly established. How long are the guests staying? Do they expect to be fed and entertained every day or will they set their own agendas? If they are staying for a while, will they make a financial contribution towards their upkeep?

Even having guests round for an evening can be stressful. How should you react if someone breaks a favorite glass or spills red wine on your cream rug? What about the drunken diehards who won't leave at four in the morning when you're dying to get to bed?

You don't want to lose any friendships or fall out with your family, but it is important that you make your boundaries quite clear from the outset.

Hired Help/Tradesmen

"In every age and clime we see
Two of a trade can never agree."

John Gay

Few of us can get through life without hiring the services of professional contractors, whether it be the caterers hired to produce a first-rate meal for your daughter's wedding or the builders called in to repaint your brickwork or an electrician to rewire your house—at some stage in your life you will need to pay for help.

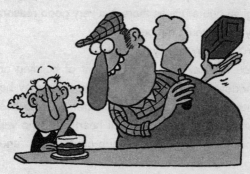

This relationship can become very stressful if each party is not fully briefed as to the other's expectations. And because money is involved, usually quite large amounts, the relationship can become more stressful still. Tales of builders arriving just before lunch time and knocking off just after four o'clock— and billing for a full day's work are plentiful. And what if the work turns out to be substandard?

STRESSBUSTERS

- Wherever possible get recommendations from friends. If you have to hire a company chosen from the telephone directory check that they are a registered member of the relevant professional association.
- Draw up a plan of action which both you and the contractors are happy with.
- Get a full quote for the job. Make it clear that any extras that crop up will have to be covered by the original quote unless there is a very good reason why they should not be.
- Don't pay any money up front.
- If you are having a large amount of building or remodeling work done on your home it may be worth employing a general contractor, who has your interests and budget at heart and who will coordinate the various sub-contractors and

---

report back to you. That way you only have to deal with one person.

- If things go wrong and you need to make a complaint, do so in writing, listing your points systematically. Contact your local Better Business Bureau or the relevant professional association if you are still not satisfied.

Holidays/Vacations

Do you feel on the verge of exhaustion when you are about to go on vacation? One of the biggest mistakes many of us make before going on vacation is to work furiously in the weeks beforehand, stop to pack a few hours before we are due to take off, pick up a few essentials and race for the airport. When we eventually arrive at our destination we collapse in an exhausted heap, and consequently spend most of our vacation asleep.

Once you reach the vacation destination, you may have to deal with one or all of the following stressful situations: communicating in a foreign language (or by sign language); unfamiliar food, money, traffic regulations and customs; and, depending on the country, you may have to take precautions against insect bites, stomach upsets and other dangers.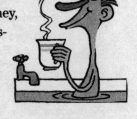

Many people have unreal expectations of vacations.

STRESSBUSTERS

- Check six weeks in advance if any vaccinations are required for your chosen destination.
- In the two weeks running up to your vacation, start to wind down to ensure that you are as relaxed as possible when you go:

  - keep pre-holiday weekends as activity-free as possible
  - aim to get better quality sleep: add six drops of lavender oil to your bath; go to bed half an hour earlier than usual; avoid drinking coffee or tea at the end of the day; drink an herbal tea, such as chamomile, instead.

- Don't leave it until midnight of the night before you go away to start looking for your passport and driver's license.
- Make contingency plans, especially if you have children.
- Do your homework—will there be plenty to keep the kids amused even if rain forces everyone inside?
- Don't pressurize yourself to make this the best vacation ever.
- Plan some time for yourself so that you can recharge your batteries.

If you are traveling out of season, check what the weather is likely to be and choose a destination with other attractions besides a beach. If you are traveling with friends or family, make sure you agree about the type of vacation before you book. Your long-awaited break could turn into a living hell if you don't plan properly.

Home Repairs

In recent years Do-it-yourself (DIY) has become more popular than ever before, and the growth of DIY superstores has encouraged many of us to attempt to repair and redecorate our own homes. While the results may be highly satisfying the process can be deeply stressful—especially if your skills fall short of the task you have set yourself. Depending on the size of the project you may find yourself knee-deep in tools and materials for weeks or months with little or no idea of how to proceed.

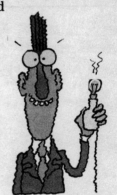

STRESSBUSTERS

• Planning and preparation are the key to successful do-it-yourself:

- do your research
- know your limitations. Hire people to do the more complicated work such as plastering, plumbing, roofing and electrical work.

- If you are completely remodeling your home, remember to keep a dust- and clutter-free room where you can relax.
- Plan for DIY-free days – this way you'll return to the project with renewed enthusiasm.

Housework

"There was no need to do any housework at all. After the first four years the dirt doesn't get any worse."

Quentin Crisp

Today when many women have to split their time between full- or part-time work and the demanding jobs of wife and/or mother, housework can seem impossible to keep up with at times.

Other people become perfectionist about housework to the extent that they feel stressed if they don't

v a c u u m
twice a day
and disinfect
surfaces regu-
larly. If this
sounds like
you, it may be
worth examin-

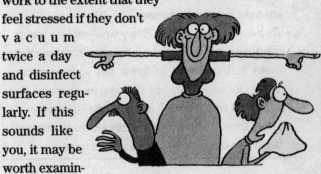

ing your obsession with cleanliness, as it is causing you unnecessary stress.

STRESSBUSTERS

- Get organized:

    - work out what needs to be done and divide the tasks between the household. To do this effectively you, your roommate, spouse, and/or family members need to make a list of occasional, daily, weekly and monthly chores.
    - assign chores by the week and draw up a list of who does what and when.
    - rotate tasks so that no one gets permanently stuck with the worst tasks.

- Consider hiring outside help for certain tasks such as window-cleaning.
- Put things where you can find them. Looking for things is one of the most time-consuming and stressful household chores.
- Throw away your clutter. Every time you buy something new, get rid of something old. This does not mean that you have to throw out your wedding dress, for example, but it does mean carefully packing it and storing it in the garage or attic.
- From time to time have a break from chores. Schedule in free time to use as you want.

Illness

Living with chronic illness or long-term pain is incredibly stressful and debilitating. It can disrupt your sleep, make you depressed and cause you to clench your muscles to avoid putting pressure on painful areas. Long-term illness places a huge burden on relationships, too. In many cases your friend and lover has to become a care-giver.

STRESSBUSTERS

- Keep a pain diary to help you plot when your good and bad times are. This will enable you to plan in activities for your "good" days.
- Fill up your time as much as possible to keep your mind off the pain.
- Use relaxation and visualization techniques to help you control the pain (see pp. 197–213).
- For chronic illnesses, it is important to pace your recovery; pushing yourself too hard can result in a relapse.
- Seek support from your friends and family.

The relationship between pain and physical damage is not fully understood. But what is known is that if you are frightened, depressed, angry or anxious these emotions will worsen your pain. Conversely, if you are happy and active, the pain lessens.

Leaving Home

"The only lasting things we can give our children are roots and wings."

Hodding Carter

A child leaving home is a stressful experience for all concerned. For parents who have prepared their offspring for leaving the nest it can be a time of mixed emotions—relief on one hand and sadness on the other. Making the move as successful as possible involves emotional and practical preparation on both sides.

As the end of adolescence approaches many young people will be looking forward to leaving home and the freedom it offers. But some will shy away from the responsibilities and hard work that this entails.

Whether your children leave home as soon as they can or put it off for as long as possible, with your blessing or in the wake of arguments, amid success or failure, is largely in the hands of the parents.

If you are the kind of parents that do everything for

your children, when they eventually leave home they may find it very difficult to make their way. Rather than thanking you for having made their years at home so comfortable, they may end up resenting you for not having properly prepared them for the outside world. Or they may even find life at home so pleasant that they never want to leave.

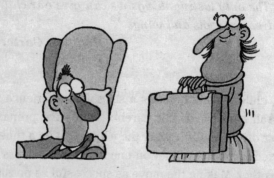

If your children show no signs of leaving home, you may have to nudge them towards the door. There is nothing wrong in suggesting that it is time that they start looking after themselves.

Once they have moved out, remember that their home is not your home. Whatever your involvement in your child's new house or apartment—you may have helped them find it, you may pay the rent or mortgage, you may even have furnished it—it does not give you the right to walk in at any time and rearrange the kitchen cupboards. This invasion of their space is likely to be met with annoyance or anger (*see also* **Parents**).

STRESSBUSTERS

- Let your children know that you expect them to leave home. It's important to present your anticipation in a positive way—for them and yourself.

- Make your children aware of how much organization and money is needed to set up house. Don't let them think that clean clothes and hot meals simply appear out of thin air. The first few months in their new home will be hellish if the everyday items they took for granted aren't on hand when they need them, and the money to pay for them has already been spent on going out and buying clothes.

- Know when to offer advice and when to stand back. They may make mistakes but at least they will feel in control of their own lives. As parents you should make it clear that you are a resource that your children can call on whenever they feel they need to.

- Once your children have left home don't be tempted to take over their new-found responsibilities for them. This will not help them adapt to the stresses of adult life in the long term.

Miscarriage

A miscarriage is the loss of a pregnancy before 20 weeks' gestation. Around 15 percent of all recognized pregnancies miscarry and as many as 25 percent of all pregnant women experience "spontaneous miscarriages" within the first two weeks of conception, but these are rarely recognized.

Losing a pregnancy can be a devastating experience. Feelings of shock and grief may be accompanied by a feeling of disorientation as the couple realize how much planning and energy they had been putting into the baby's arrival.

There are many factors that can lead to a miscarriage, ranging from physical preconditions to environmental hazards.

- Genetic problems are the main cause of spontaneous miscarriages, accounting for 55 percent.
- A miscarriage is twice as likely to occur in women over 34 as in women under 30.
- Smoking is the most common environmental hazard linked to miscarriage. Smokers are

25 percent more likely to miscarry than non-smokers. Alcohol and illicit drugs have a similar risk. Women who smoke heavily and/or consume more than 1 or 2 servings of alcohol a week and/or recreational drugs are more likely to have a poor nutritional intake, which can contribute to a miscarriage.

Miscarriage will also be stressful and upsetting for your partner, although he doesn't have any physical symptoms to deal with. It is important for your relationship that you are able to discuss your feelings openly—these may include guilt, anger and frustration, as well as grief.

STRESSBUSTERS

- Try not to worry unduly. A single miscarriage does not necessarily affect your chances of having a successful pregnancy in the future.
- Give your body a good chance to rest and recover after miscarriage before trying to conceive again. Most experts advise at least four to six months between pregnancies to allow hormone levels to stabilize.
- Don't smoke, eat a well balanced diet, exercise gently, don't lift heavy objects, and consult your doctor about taking vitamins.
- Talk to other women who have miscarried.

- Complementary therapies such as herbalism and acupuncture, which help to rebalance your body, may be worth looking into if you have had more than one miscarriage. And an aromatherapy massage will help ease your anxiety.

Money

"Always try to rub up against money."

Damon Runyon

Financial difficulties are one of the biggest causes of stress, and arguments about money are one of the main causes of relationship break-ups. Money can also affect friendships. While a friend will probably tell us how good her new lover is in bed, we won't have a clue how much he earns. The secrecy that surrounds money often makes us feel guilty and envious of what other people earn and can poison friendships.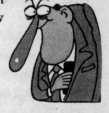

Managing your money well means being clear about what you want from your life, making realistic plans and controlling your expenditures. If you owe money, work out the size of your total debt and then how much money you have left after all the bills have been paid. Discuss the situation with your partner or family, then start to economize. Creditors will be more inclined to help if you answer their letters. If you have a mortgage, talk to your lender and discuss the possibility of stopping or reducing payment for a time. Debts left unresolved can threaten the way you live, your home and your family. Whatever the cause of your money problems, you cannot leave the responsibility of sorting them out to someone else.

STRESSBUSTERS

- Keep a diary of all your finances—what you have in the bank as savings and insurance policies.
- Keep a record of your expenditures—down to the last penny. After a week or so, you will be able to pinpoint where you are frittering away your money.
- File all your financial documents in a safe place.
- Keep an emergency fund, if possible, to help you through lean times.
- Pay off credit cards regularly. Beware of special deals.
- If you have accumulated more credit card debt than you can handle:

    - cut up your cards or give them to a reliable friend for safekeeping and concentrate on paying off the balance.

- only take a debit card or cash when you go shopping.
- ask the company to lower your limit, so that you can't charge anything new.

• For advice on dealing with serious debt problems, contact your local consumer credit counseling service.

Moving

Whether you are buying or renting a new home the moving process is nearly always stressful. Dealing with landlords, banks, lawyers and real estate agents to secure your new home is difficult enough in itself, and then comes the act of physically moving yourself, your family and all your belongings from one place to another. Good planning is a key strategy in keeping moving-day stress levels as low as possible.

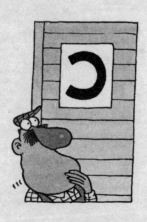

STRESSBUSTERS

- Make floor plans of your new home and decide where you want large items of furniture to go. Give the moving company a copy of this plan.
- Allocate a number or letter to each room in the new house, and mark boxes with corresponding letters to show where each box should go. List the contents of each box on a separate sheet of paper so you can find the most essential items quickly.
- If you are using a moving company let them do your packing for you.

Parents

*"Children aren't happy with nothing to ignore,
And that's what parents were created for."*
                              Ogden Nash, **The Parents**

Do your parents insist on interfering in your life long after you left home? Some people have to deal with mothers who criticize their methods of child-rearing or complain that they haven't produced grandchildren yet; others have fathers who offer unsolicited advice on everything from home repairs to careers, new car purchases and the way they dress.

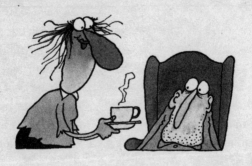

Maybe you welcome your parents' advice but for some people it can become very irritating and stressful. It may be that your parents no longer have enough stimulation in their own lives—perhaps they have retired and have too much time on their hands. Try to be patient if you can—one day the advice or help they offer may be exactly what you need.

STRESSBUSTERS

For those looking after an elderly relative:

- Develop good assertiveness skills.
- Maintain your own friends.
- Arrange time alone with your family.
- Take regular breaks and holidays on your own.
- Arrange for practical and financial support.
- Share the responsibility with the rest of the family.
- You don't have to be perfect; it is common to feel guilty and lose your temper or feel embarrassed by your elderly parents' odd behavior.

As we get older the question of caring for our parents becomes a more pressing concern. Around 20 percent of the population are of retirement age. Of these, 6 percent are in institutions and the rest are looked after by a huge network of care-givers many of whom are unpaid family members.

Deciding how to look after a parent whose mental

and/or physical abilities may be deteriorating is a difficult one. The relative merits of moving them into a residential home, or to a smaller home close enough for you to pop in most days, or moving them into your own house need to be carefully considered. The last option will obviously have the biggest impact on your life and that of your partner and children. If you feel that you are the best person to look after an elderly parent and want them living either with or near you, you will need to ensure that you don't forget to look after yourself.

Partners

Meeting and falling in love with someone is a blissfully happy time. Translating that initial magic into a happy relationship means being able to adapt and share your life with another person whose views you take into account alongside your own.

When the initial passion and fire die away, just how well your partnership matures depends on a number of factors: respect and liking for each other, a shared sense of humor, common interests, complementary personalities and mutual physical attraction.

Typical relationship stressors can include:

- lack of self-love or self-understanding
- "make me happy" partner dependency
- poor communication
- past patterns upsetting present relationships
- not enough quality "together time"

- being judgmental
- different sexual needs
- no common purpose or direction
- failure to show love and respect
- an unequal share of responsibility

STRESSBUSTERS

- Know yourself. If you are to be comfortable with another person, it helps to be at ease with yourself first.
- Talk to each other. When communication fails the relationship fails.
- Show the real you. If you want your relationship to be honest and true, then you owe it to yourself and your partner to express the real you.
- Listen to each other. Too often we can be too busy making a point, allocating blame or assuming too much to listen properly to what the other person is saying. The biggest mistake you can make is to believe that you already listen enough. There is nearly always something new to hear.
- Respect each other. Egos are delicate and sensitive things that require all the love, understanding and respect we can give them.
- Discuss your expectations: good relations can be swamped by what is usually an unspoken contract of expectations which the other person has to somehow instinctively know and live up to.

- Accept responsibility for your relationship.
- Personal space—or the lack of it—can be a huge source of stress in relationships. Both partners must appreciate the importance of personal time and space.

Phobias

"I have three phobias . . . I hate to go to bed, I hate to get up, and I hate to be alone."

Tallulah Bankhead

A phobia is defined as an irrational persistent fear of a particular thing or situation.

Mild phobias affect more than one in ten people at some time in their lives and are often caused by a traumatic incident. But, more often than not they are caused when we start to avoid situations that make us anxious. This avoidance behavior can lower stress levels but only in the short term. Then, the next time we come up against the same situation our anxiety will be even greater. If a phobia is not tackled it can begin to interfere with daily life.

There are three types of phobia: simple, social and complex.

1. Simple phobias center on one specific thing or situation. A fear of dogs or spiders, snakes, mice, heights, darkness, lightning, blood and needles are all simple phobias.
2. A social phobia is a fear of meeting new people, eating with others, public speaking, or other social situations.
3. Complex phobias are more stressful and disabling in that they combine a number of fears and intense panic attacks. Agoraphobics, in addition to their fear of leaving the house, commonly fear crowded shops, buses, elevators, heights and enclosed spaces.

Simple phobias are, as their name suggests, relatively easy to resolve. The most common treatment involves controlled or graded exposure to the anxiety-causing situation or object. By progressively confronting that fear, anxiety diminishes and recovery follows. Graded exposure is also helpful for people with complex phobias, especially agoraphobics.

If your phobia is restricting your life, seek help from a doctor or counselor. Hypnotherapy (*see* pp. 195–96) can also be effective in the treatment of phobias.

STRESSBUSTERS

- Get to grips with where your fear came from—is it linked to a bad experience or an unresolved fear from your childhood?
- Write down what you think will happen to you if you face your fear.
- Practice some relaxation exercises (*see* pp.197–209).

Pregnancy

The decision to have a baby is a momentous one for a couple. But it can be an extremely hard one to make because there is rarely a perfect time. You may be trying to climb a few more rungs up the career ladder before you take time out. You may have taken on financial commitments, such as a large mortgage, and worry how you'll manage without your income. Maybe the pregnancy wasn't planned and you need some time to come to terms with it.

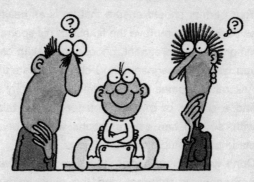

Nobody can ever fully anticipate how they will feel or cope once pregnancy is a reality. To ensure your pregnancy is as stress-free as possible, don't forget your partner. He will be as bewildered as you by the changes taking place, so keep him involved. Be tolerant and look after each other.

STRESSBUSTERS

- Before you conceive, get your doctor to check your immunity against rubella (German measles). Start taking 400mg of folic acid daily, to reduce the risk of spina bifida.

- Get in the best of health. If you smoke, give it up. If you are overweight, try to lose the extra weight before conception or you will be more likely to experience problems during the pregnancy. Start exercising in order to make your muscles supple and eat a nutritious, balanced diet.

- Your partner should ensure that he is as healthy as possible, to improve the fitness of his sperm.

- When you are pregnant, choose the health care you want for pregnancy and childbirth carefully. Ask other women for recommendations. Try to find a doctor or midwife you feel comfortable with, so you can ask questions without being made to feel stupid or over-anxious.

- Don't worry about horror stories you hear. Every pregnancy is different and the overwhelming probability is that yours will go smoothly and you will have a beautiful, healthy baby at the end of it.

INFERTILITY

If you experience problems getting pregnant, there are a number of techniques you can try before opting for full medical intervention:

• Be as relaxed as possible about trying for a baby. Stress is one of the biggest inhibitors of fertility.
• You are fertile for the week before ovulation until the day afterwards. Ovulation occurs approximately mid-cycle, with your period coming 14 days later. But take other factors into consideration—if you have a busy job, other children to look after, a partner with an equally hectic lifestyle, the last thing you want to feel is pressurized to have sex at the right biological time but wrong emotional time.
• If you have been trying unsuccessfully for a year to become pregnant, this is the time to ask your doctor to refer you for fertility investigations.
• Traditional Chinese medicine may also be effective in treating fertility problems.

Public Speaking

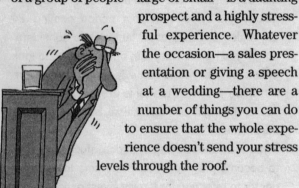

or many people the thought of standing up in front of a group of people—large or small—is a daunting prospect and a highly stressful experience. Whatever the occasion—a sales presentation or giving a speech at a wedding—there are a number of things you can do to ensure that the whole experience doesn't send your stress levels through the roof.

STRESSBUSTERS

- Prepare yourself: try the speech out beforehand on a guinea pig and time yourself.
- Summarize your speech on index cards.
- Keep the structure simple and speak slowly.

- If you are going to be using any technical equipment check that it will all be on hand when you need it and, if possible, try it out beforehand.
- Have a glass of water nearby.
- Go for a brisk walk a few hours beforehand to encourage the release of calming substances called endorphins.

Reduction/
Unemployment

*"After Cambridge—unemployment. No one
much wanted to know. Good degrees are good
for nothing in the business world below."*
Gavin Ewart, The Sentimental Education

The notion of a job for life has well and truly gone.
With so many people out of work
the prospect of unemployment is
one that is faced by both the
unskilled and professional worker
alike. Studies have found that being
out of work affects workers
from all areas of the job market in similar ways causing:

- unhappiness
- dissatisfaction with life
- low self-esteem

- increased depression
- poor concentration

STRESSBUSTERS

- Make finding a job your job. Try to view the situation as a challenge. Make a list of your strengths to help you to sell yourself at your next interview. These may include:

  - knowledge
  - experience
  - skills
  - natural abilities.

- Give yourself time to find a new job.
- Plan things to fill your day, even if it's a trip to the library or the local swimming pool, or a matinee performance at the cinema.
- Learn a new skill by enrolling in an evening class.
- Try to keep yourself physically fit—this will help you to stay active and feeling positive.
- Don't let your appearance go just because you're not going into work each day. Looking good will also help you to you feel good about yourself.

Research has also found that there is a strong link between physical illness and unemployment-related stress. Studies have found that unemployed people report significantly more symptoms of bronchitis, ear, nose and throat problems, and allergies than those employed.

If unemployment happens to you, it is important not to dwell in the past, looking for what went wrong, but move forward and try to keep yourself optimistic and motivated.

Retirement

After a lifetime of hard work, going into retirement can be a stressful time. It can mean the change from being a key player in an important organization and making a valuable contribution to society, to a position where your usefulness in the world seems to have been stripped away from you.

The most commonly experienced retirement-related stresses are:

- boredom: worrying what to do with your time
- loneliness and isolation
- lack of purpose: no clear sense of direction
- money worries

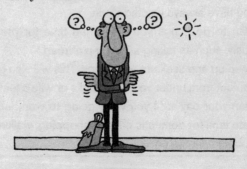

● poor self-confidence: the need for a new self-image and a new place in society

But it's not as if you don't see it coming. Unlike downsizing and sudden unemployment, you can plan for your retirement, both in terms of financial security and keeping yourself occupied.

STRESSBUSTERS

- As the time for your retirement approaches, cut back your hours gradually so that you don't go straight from full-time employment to full-time unemployment.
- If you can't face the prospect of having no work at all think about taking a part-time job or doing volunteer work for a charity, but take care not to let your life become as stressful as it was pre-retirement.
- Use your free time to take up a hobby, or enroll in a continuing-education class to learn something you have always wanted to do.
- Plan to do things you never had time for previously, such as taking a long trip abroad.
- Keep up and seek out old friends. This will also get you out from under your husband's or wife's feet.
- Plan your day as if you were going to work: allocate time for domestic chores, shopping, walking, hobbies and so on.

Road Rage

"The car has become the carapace, the protective and aggressive shell, of urban and suburban man."

Marshall McLuhan

The phrase "road rage" may strictly speaking be a 1990s one, but the concept it describes is not new. The frustration experienced by a motorist driving in congested traffic or by one who has come to a halt in a ten-mile back-up has been around just about as long as the motor car itself. And these days both men and women drivers are as likely to "cut off" or abuse other drivers.

The ever-increasing volume of traffic means it is unlikely that driving will get any easier. Whether you are sitting in rush-hour traffic or taking your family out for the day over a three-day holiday weekend, driving can cause the symptoms of stress—the release of adrenaline, accelerated heartbeat, higher blood pressure and so on—that can lead to an explosion of emotion now known as road rage.

Aggressive drivers vastly increase the risk of accidents—for themselves and everyone else in the vicinity. Resist the temptation to use your horn or to retaliate if someone cuts in front of you. People in this aggressive state can be dangerous. Remember the media reports of incidents that turned into full-scale attacks and even murders, and whatever you do don't stop and get out of the car to remonstrate personally with the other driver. Do your best to get out of the way of an aggressive driver, even if it means pulling onto the side of the road to let him or her by.

See also **Cars, Driving.**

STRESSBUSTERS
- Build in extra time for delays.
- If you do get caught up in traffic, accept the situation. Allowing your stress level to rise won't get you moving any faster.
- The music you listen to while driving can affect your performance. Whether classical or pop, music above 60 beats per minute increases your heart rate and blood pressure. Avoid Wagner's *Ride of the Valkyries* and Motorhead's *Ace of*

Spades; listen to The Beatles' *Here Comes the Sun* or Bach's *Cello Suite No. 1*.

- Meditate or practice a simple relaxation exercise (*see* pp. 175–82).
- Avoid eye contact with other drivers and don't be fooled by age—older people in suits can be just as likely to be violent as younger drivers in jeans.

School

Today's children lead quite stressful lives. And, like adults, they often suffer the consequences emotionally and physically. For some inner-city children, just getting to school each day can be stressful in itself. Then, once at school they face the pressure of making friends, fitting in or being bullied. The latter is something that many children feel ashamed of or too scared to admit to their teachers or parents.

It is not always easy for parents and teachers to know when children are under stress at school but there are some signs:

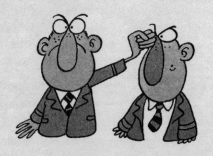

- Bad behavior and unusually poor schoolwork are often signs that something is wrong.
- When a child suddenly becomes quiet and withdrawn, and passes up activities that would normally interest him, this can be a sign of depression. (Depression can affect children as young as eight, but the risks increase with age. Given the high incidence of teenage suicides, getting immediate professional help is vital.)

Exams are also a source of stress for most school children and particularly for those high-achievers who are expected to do well.

See **Exams and Tests.**

STRESSBUSTERS

To help your children through school days:

- give them regular meals and healthy snacks to keep up their blood sugar levels.
- encourage periods of exercise and relaxation-however short.
- make sure they get enough sleep.
- take an interest in and supervise homework to make sure it doesn't turn into an unmanageable burden.
- offer to help them draw up a revision timetable.
- encourage the whole family to be supportive.

- make sure they have a quiet, comfortable place to work.
- don't add pressure by expressing your hopes or fears about results.
- don't give extra coffee or tea—stimulants such as caffeine can contribute to stress.
- ask how they are getting along with their teachers.
- ask if they have any special friends or if there are any children they don't get along with or who scare them.

Sex

"The best way to talk about what you want in bed is out of bed."

Wendy Bristow

Talking about sex is a tricky business. But given that not many couples spot each other across the room, leap into bed and hit the bull's-eye from the beginning, the only way to get the kind of sex you want is to show or tell your partner.

The difficulty is how to talk to your partner with-

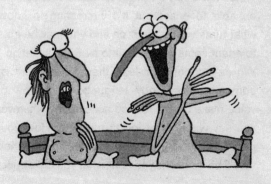

out shattering their delicate ego. However well you know them, saying "This is what I like and this is what I don't like" will feel like a criticism that goes straight to where they feel most vulnerable. But at some point if you want to save your sex life and ultimately your relationship you are going to have to initiate a conversation about your love life.

STRESSBUSTERS

- Talk about the behavior not the person. Instead of saying "You're terrible in bed," say "I'd really like it if you did X more often." Use positive language: say "This is how we could do this better," rather than "Here's what you are doing wrong."

- If you find it hard to talk about sex, discuss it out of bed and try to keep things quite lighthearted. Have a fun conversation about your secret fantasies, to which you both have to contribute. These need not be practical ideas that you will be able to enact but it's interesting to know what turns your partner on and you may be able to adapt some elements into a sexual situation.

- Words account for less than 10 percent of communication—body language and tone of voice make up the rest so accompany whatever you say with lots of loving touching. Hold your partner's hand and look into their eyes—then they'll be more likely to hear what you are saying.

- Always thank your partner for listening and when they do what you ask, praise them. When you are having a good time as a result or your conversation, make sure your partner knows.
- Never make fun of your partner's sexual prowess or physical attributes. Everyone is sensitive in these areas and ridicule could kill your sex life altogether.

Shopping

Shopping can be a pleasure when you have a day to devote to it. But for most people, most of the time, shopping for food and clothes is just one of many chores to be fitted into a life chock-full of things to do.

It is particularly stressful if you have to return goods that are defective to unhelpful store clerks, but make sure you know your consumer rights and insist on them.

STRESSBUSTERS

- Write out a week's menu in advance and make your shopping list from this. List things in categories: for example "dairy" will be shorthand for milk, eggs, cheese, yogurt and so on.

- If you can, shop early in the morning when the stores will be less crowded.
- Keep the things that you will need to make a meal when you get home in a separate carrier bag.
- If you have Internet access, you can order direct from some supermarkets and have them deliver to your door.

Single People

Have you got to that stage in your life when nearly all your friends are married or in long-term relationships? Is your mother making less-than-subtle hints about how she would like to cuddle a grandchild before she dies? Have your friends started trying to pair you off with their few surviving single friends? Even in these enlightened times the pressure to be part of a couple is enormous. But if you are the shy and retiring type and don't especially enjoy picking up people in nightclubs how do you set about finding a soul mate?

STRESSBUSTERS

- Join an evening class or a club.
- Make contact with old friends—they could introduce you to a new circle of friends.
- Reassess what you're looking for—it could be that you are being too choosy.

- Join a professional dating agency.
- At the next party you go to make an effort to mingle and chat with at least five new people.
- Remember that many of your friends in relationships are actually jealous of your freedom!

Technology

If you are still getting to grips with using a pocket calculator and programming your video recorder, the chances are that the thought of using a personal computer, electronic organizer, surfing the net, or sending e-mail sends a cold chill down your spine.

Technology is moving forward at a lightning pace. And if, so far, the revolution has passed you by, it's time you jumped aboard. The good news is that most computers are easier to use than they were ten years ago. And once you have cracked that techno-nut, mastering the net and e-mail will seem easy.

The bad news is that a large number of problems 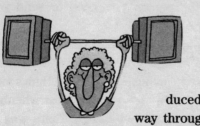 can still occur with computers. Information can get lost, viruses can be intro- duced that eat their way through your files, the machine can crash right in the middle of an important document, or your programs might be incompatible

STRESSBUSTERS

- To join the techno-revolution you need some basic training—ask a friend who works with computers to show you the ropes or sign up for a night class.
- If your employers can't send you on a computer course you should be able to join one at your local community college.
- Use the manufacturers' helplines for advice and also check how long a product is waranteed for so you can return it for repairs if necessary.
- There are many useful PC and Internet magazines available to tell you about new products.
- Buy one of the virus-protection systems on the market and update it regularly to protect your computer from viruses.
- Take screen breaks every 20 minutes.

with those of the person you need to send your work to.

Most people using computers don't understand how they work. We all learn what we need to know when we need to use it, but there are few things more stressful than the computer acting up just when you have an important deadline looming. That's why it's important to have technical support on hand (or on the other end of a telephone).

If you link up to an e-mail and Internet provider, make sure they have a screening system so that you don't receive unsolicited pornographic and other objectionable material downline. And be very wary of giving your credit card number if making purchases on the net—hackers can break into many networks and use your number themselves.

Telephoning

Just about every household these days has a telephone, but this communication box is not as warmly welcomed by some as by others. For some people, the minute they attempt to talk on the phone all rational thought flies out of their head. Incoming calls, particularly badly timed and unwanted calls, can be the bane of many people's work and personal lives.

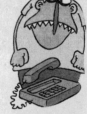

STRESSBUSTERS

- Have all your calls screened at work. In many cases, someone else will be able to supply the information the caller requires.
- If necessary, be "out of the office" rather than "in a meeting." This is far less annoying to your callers, many of whom will expect you to interrupt your meeting for them.
- Call back punctually. If you have said you will call a person back at a specific time—do it.

- If your mind goes to mush on the phone, make a list of what you want to say and keep it nearby.
- Avoid having long conversations on your mobile phone, especially while driving.

Unforeseen Circumstances

"Habit is a great deadener."
Samuel Beckett, Waiting for Godot

In life there are probably only two certainties: the sun will rise in the east and set in the west. Yet most of us plan our lives as if we know exactly how each and every step will pan out.

Rather like accidents, unforeseen circumstances are stressful precisely because they are unexpected. We are creatures of habit and, as far as possible, we like to know where our lives are heading. At the start of every new year, we make resolutions for where we would like to be and what we would like to achieve by the end of it.

Depending on their magnitude, unforeseen circumstances can be rather like having the rug pulled out from under your feet, leaving you at the very least feeling disoriented and confused and at worst, undermining long-held values and beliefs. But rather than throw your hands up in despair, try to take time to consider how to make the best of a new situation, which could bring exciting new opportunities.

STRESSBUSTERS

- Be flexible and be prepared to drop routines.
- Give up the need for absolute control—if you are prepared to trust that life will bring you what you need, most crises will pass far more easily.
- Live in the present, not the future.
- Don't get bogged down by too many details—focus on the broader picture.
- Be grateful for what you have now; this will help you to weather major upheavals calmly and with dignity.
- Step out of your comfort zone: push the boundaries of life back a little so you don't get too comfortable or too complacent. That way, when the unexpected happens, the shock to your system is lessened.

University/College

For many people, going to college is also the time when they leave home. It's a period of great excitement, fear and insecurity all rolled into one. You are not only coming to grips with a new environment, but also striving to make new friends and cope with a new level of learning. Having reached the top of the pecking order in high 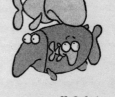 school you may suddenly feel like a very small fish in an extremely large, cold pond.

STRESSBUSTERS

- Go to the freshman fair. All the college clubs and societies will be there trying to sign up new members and these are an ideal way of meeting potential new friends with similar interests.
- Don't sit next to the same person in lectures—move around. That way you'll get a better feeling for the type of people in your major.

- Strike up conversations with people as you wait for lectures or line up in the dining hall. Smile and don't be afraid to be yourself.
- Manage your coursework. If you have to write an essay or a project that seems overwhelming, break it up into manageable chunks—research, planning, reading, writing—and do a bit at a time.

Work

"Around 183,000 people in the UK experience stress and depression caused or made worse by work."

Health Education Authority

Stress at work can stem from a general sense of vulnerability about how long you can expect to stay in the job. With downsizing almost commonplace, jobs for life are a thing of the past. In larger firms, this sense of unease can be compounded by

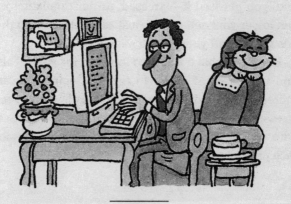

poor communication channels which feed the rumor mill rather than providing constructive information about what is happening.

Other work stresses can include having to negotiate your own pay raise. Go armed with good reasons why you should receive the amount you are asking for but be prepared to be flexible as well. Being promoted or passed over for promotion each bring new pressures: a bigger workload and new responsibilities or a blow to your self-confidence. While the latter may feel like the end of the world, the key is not to get too anxious and make contingency plans.

For women, returning to work after having your family can be very stressful. If you're worried that your skills may be a little rusty, ask your local authority about courses for women returnees.

A stress-free job may seem like heaven, but too little stress can leave you feeling demotivated, bored and, you guessed it—stressed. An unstimulating job can lower your self-esteem just as surely as a job that has you run off your feet.

Employers have a duty to look out for your health and happiness at work. In the U.S. employers are increasingly held responsible for their employees' stress-related health problems. And in the UK bosses who expose their staff to severe stress could soon face prosecution.

STRESSBUSTERS

- Recognizing those parts of your job that are most stressful is the first step. Make a list of all the elements your job involves: your workload—too much or too little? Is there too much travel? Is your working day too long? Give each a score from 0–5 to help you to see which areas of your job are a problem.
- Don't regularly take work home.
- Keep your working hours reasonable.
- Don't be a perfectionist—just do the best you can.
- Delegate; you don't have to do everything yourself.
- Divide overwhelming tasks into 20-minute blocks.
- Say no to interruptions; find a quiet place to work.
- Personalize your workspace with photos, pictures or plants.
- Keep a stress diary; this will provide you with information about the type of situation or person that causes you the most problems.
- Manage your time: list your tasks for the day, number them in order of priority and stick to the order where possible. But be flexible too.
- Take regular breaks every 20 minutes or so to help you maintain your concentration.

But you should still take personal responsibility for your own stress levels and take action to deal with them if life is becoming unbearable. See also the tips in **Bosses, Colleagues** and **Discrimination** and check your **Stress Rating** score (*see* pp. 32–3) from time to time to ensure you are not putting your health at risk.

Quick Tips for Beating Stress

BREATHE IT OUT

When we are stressed, angry or frightened one of the first things that happens is that our breathing pattern changes. Our breathing becomes quick, shallow and irregular. The medical term for this breathing pattern is "hyperventilation" or over-breathing. Some people over-breathe without realizing it. This pattern often begins as a result of a shock or fear but, once you become aware of it, can lead to more worry and anxiety.

People who are worried about their breathing are usually concerned about getting enough fresh air and oxygen. But the rate and depth of our breathing is influenced not by a lack of oxygen but by the amount of carbon dioxide in the blood. When we over-breathe we take in more oxygen than the body needs and expel too much carbon dioxide. This alters the acidity of the blood, causing dizziness, shaking, tension, or sweating and it may cause a sense of panic.

Acute over-breathing is the cause of most panic attacks. Controlling your breathing—by slowing it down, using the lower part of the lungs and focusing on letting all the air out of your lungs—is often the first step towards successful stress control. To be relaxed it is important to allow your breathing to be relaxed too.

Here are some simple breathing-control exercises to use when you are in a stressful situation.

BREATHE INTO A PAPER BAG

If you are having a panic attack, breathe hard into a paper bag and rebreathe the carbon-dioxide-rich air that you have just exhaled. If you don't have a bag, cup your hands together and place them over your nose. Do not repeat more than five times.

DON'T GULP FOR AIR

If you are feeling anxious and are aware of your breathing becoming more rapid and shallow, don't gulp for more air. Slowly breathe out as much as you can then let the air into your lungs without effort.

BREATHE EASY

Breathe deeply and slowly, focusing on each breath as you inhale and exhale, and you will become calm.

COUNT IT OUT

Repeat the following exercise until your breathing pattern becomes more regular and smooth:

- Breathe in for a count of four.
- Breathe out for a count of four.
- Pause for a count of four.

SHUT YOUR MOUTH

If you are so panicked that it is hard to catch your breath, you need to stop hyperventilating by exhaling; empty your lungs completely and expel old air.

Close your mouth. Put one hand on your abdomen just above your navel. Breathe in through your nose, slowly counting to three. Try to make the breath push your hand up. Pause for a second, then exhale, this time to a count of four. The out breath is longer to enable you to fully empty your lungs on each breath and this will stop you taking short, panicky breaths.

When you start to feel calmer, slow your breathing even more by inhaling to a count of four, pause, and exhaling for a count of five. Practice for at least three minutes.

THE EFFECTS OF POOR BREATHING

- the body is robbed of nourishment
- the nervous system is weakened
- energy is sapped
- muscle tension occurs
- blood pressure increases or decreases
- circulation is blocked
- digestion is upset
- the immune system is undermined

Note: With all these breathing control exercises it is important to practice in advance so that when you next feel anxious you'll know exactly what to do.

STRESS RELIEVERS

Here are some simple techniques you can use in everyday situations:

MUSCLE TENSION

The following exercise is useful when you are in a stressful situation from which you can't escape, such as a meeting. It helps to burn up the stress hormones flowing around your body:

Tighten up every muscle in your body as hard as you can. Hold and then let go and relax. Repeat until you find yourself relaxing.

REALITY TESTING

This is an effective exercise that works on the fact that your body can't focus on two things at the same time. By forcing you to pay attention to the environment around you, it helps you to calm down:

Say out loud, to yourself, five things you can see, hear or feel. Repeat four or five times until you feel calmer and more in control.

WALK AWAY

When you feel angry or stressed, go for a brisk ten-minute walk. Head for a park or go into the garden.

TALK IT OUT

Empty your stresses out of your head and into the open by chatting to someone you trust. Articulating your problems often takes you halfway to solving them.

HAVE A GOOD STRETCH

Symptoms of mental stress can often lead to muscular tension, especially if you have been sitting at a desk for most of the day. The following workout can be done sitting at your desk. Practice it at least once a day during your lunchtime or whenever you begin to feel tense.

1. Sit up straight in your chair with your bottom pushed well into the base of the chair and your feet flat on the floor. Keeping your back straight, stretch your arms out behind you as far as you can. Raise your arms as high as possible for a count of ten. Relax and repeat.

2. Still sitting in the same position, hold your arms out straight in front of you at shoulder height. Turn your palms away from your body as if you were pushing against a wall, and push from your shoulders. Hold for a count of ten. Relax and repeat.

3. Still sitting upright hold on to the sides of your chair and push your body upwards so that you

can feel your spine stretching. Imagine that you are being pulled up by a string from the top of your head. Hold for a count of ten and relax.

4. Still sitting upright, with your feet flat on the floor bend your elbows and raise your arms to shoulder height. With your palms facing towards your body, circle your right arm back five times and then forward five times. Repeat with your left arm, and relax.

5. Still sitting upright, gently move your head from side to side. First look over your left shoulder as far as you can and then look over your right shoulder. Repeat five times on each side. Then facing forward, gently drop your head sideways towards your left shoulder, and then towards your right shoulder. Repeat five times and relax.

6. Still sitting with your feet flat on the floor, stretch your arms up towards the ceiling as far as you can. With your back straight, gently stretch your spine to release the tension in your shoulders and back. Relax and shake out your arms.

7. Finish off by relaxing your whole body. Bend forward, resting your elbows and forearms on your lap, palms facing upwards. Bend your head, close your eyes and breathe deeply and evenly for one minute. Feel the tension ease out of your neck, shoulders, back, legs and feet.

CALMING SCENTS

Certain aromas activate the production of the relaxing chemical serotonin in the brain. For relief of anxiety attacks, try putting a few drops of the following aromatherapy oils on a tissue and have a good sniff when you feel your stress levels rising.

- lavender
- chamomile
- clary sage
- neroli
- jasmine
- vetiver

FLOWERS TO THE RESCUE

There are some wonderful remedies made from flowers of which the best-known, Bach Rescue Remedy, is ideal for emergencies and life's everyday stresses. Simply add four drops of the remedy to a glass of water and sip it slowly every three to five minutes until you feel better.

Alternatively, place four drops under your tongue, or rub it on your lips, temples, wrists and behind the ears. (Bear in mind the undiluted remedy contains alcohol and tastes strongly of brandy.)

There are a number of other flower remedies available for treating different types of emotional problems, from anxiety to loneliness. Check with your local health food store for details.

DE-CLUTTER YOUR DESK

If your desk looks as if a very large bomb has been dropped on it, take some time out to reorganize. Creating order out of disorder also gives you the mental and physical space to become calm.

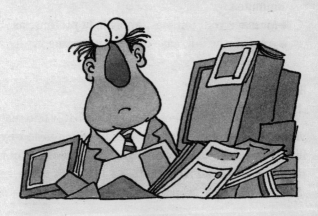

THINK POSITIVE

Talk to yourself constructively. Use affirmations— positive statements you can repeat to yourself to boost your confidence and calm you down, for example: "Every moment I feel calmer and calmer." *See* p. 222 for some other examples of affirmations.

ACUPRESSURE

Try pressing the following when you have an anxiety attack:

- With your palm facing up, use the fingers of the other hand to press a point on the little-finger side of your arm, an inch below one of your wrists. Massage in tiny circles for up to three minutes.
- Massage your temples. Apply light pressure as you breathe out, ease off as you breathe in.

RELAX YOUR JAW

When you are feeling tense you will probably find that you are clenching your jaw. Relieve this tension by lightly pushing your tongue against the roof of your mouth behind your front teeth.

BREAK THE HABIT

Many stresses and anxieties are habitual. When you feel anxious or panicky, do something you wouldn't normally do. Stand where you would normally sit and vice-versa.

PLAY SOME MUSIC

Select a favorite tape or CD with soothing melodies, sit down and listen properly. Some types of music—heavy metal, for instance—are not as suitable for this but choose whatever works for you. Keep tapes in the car, or carry a personal stereo for use outside the home.

TAKE A BREAK

If you feel your anxiety levels rising, stop whatever you are doing and do something else. Alternatively, go somewhere quiet, even if it's only the bathroom, and take a minute to gather your thoughts and work out how you are going to calm yourself down.

Relaxation Therapies

Relaxation is one of the most effective ways to free yourself from the damaging effects of long-term stress. There are a number of very successful techniques for achieving a fully relaxed state. Try any of the following that appeal to you:

MASSAGE

Massage is one of the most effective antidotes to stress. It relaxes and revitalizes the body and mind and it is particularly good at treating anxiety, tension and stress-related conditions.

While stress is a relatively new phenomenon, this therapy is centuries old. Its first recorded use dates back to 3000 BC. Massage is a natural extension of our need to touch and be touched. It was used in Chinese, Japanese, Indian and Egyptian medicine. Massage used to be an integral part of family life—used to soothe crying babies, ease painful limbs and comfort the distressed. In Europe massage treatment gained popularity in the 19th century, when Swedish gymnast Per Henrik Ling developed the strokes of what we now call Swedish massage.

Many of today's diseases may be attributable to stress and tension. Repressed emotions, which some therapists believe are held in the muscles of the body, can be released through the kneading and stroking movements of massage. During a treatment session a therapist will devise a program to suit individual needs. It could be a light relaxing massage or something much deeper.

Just how effective massage is seems to depend not only on the skill of the person administering the treatment but the reaction of the client. If the therapist is relaxed and focused on giving you the best possible treatment, the benefits to the client will be more than physical. Equally, during a deep tissue massage, if the client tenses up—perhaps because an area feels tender or painful—this will counteract any benefits. It is important to take long, deep breaths which will help relaxation, and so improve the quality of the treatment.

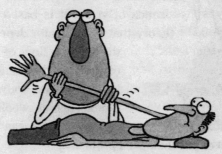

Massage should not be thought of as a luxury. Clinics and beauty salons advertise different charges, so shop around. Also many local health clubs offer massage treatment. If you feel that an hour on a massage couch is too time-consuming, opt for a back, neck and shoulder treatment which only takes about 15–30 minutes. Also there is an increasing number of on-site massage companies who can give you a treatment while you are at your desk.

In addition to the basic Swedish massage, a number of different massage treatments is available. Why not try a few and see which one you like best?

SHIATSU

Shiatsu, which means finger pressure, is a relatively new branch of Oriental medicine. It was developed in Japan at the beginning of the 20th century, but it stems from Chinese medicine which goes back thousands of years. It is based on the theory that good health depends on the smooth flow of energy (or "chi," as the Chinese call it) around the body. When block-ages or weaknesses interrupt this flow, it can lead to physical or psychological problems.

The chi is said to flow along energy pathways called meridians, which form a network all over the body. Shiatsu practitioners learn to feel blockages in the meridians. They use their fingers, palms, elbows, arms, knees and feet to apply pressure to and massage the meridians to release any blockages. Patients do not get undressed for Shiatsu treatment.

THAI MASSAGE

This vigorous massage, which is performed while you are fully clothed, can make you feel as though you have just had a workout at the gym. The therapist works on the thumbs, elbows and feet of patients to release tension and blockages in energy channels that criss-cross the body. This type of massage is ideal for people who don't get much exercise, as it helps to increase flexibility and mobility.

TUI-NA

A form of Chinese massage, this is similar to, but more vigorous than, shiatsu. As with shiatsu, the client remains clothed, and the practitioner works on the muscles, joints and the body's energy system. Tui-na is used to aid relaxation, and relieve pain and treat musculo-skeletal conditions, such as neck and shoulder problems and sciatica.

AYURVEDIC MASSAGE

Therapists use simple strokes to help rebalance the mind and body. Problems such as anxiety, insomnia, high blood pressure, respiratory and digestive conditions can all benefit from regular treatment.

INDIAN HEAD MASSAGE

Practiced in India for more than a thousand years, this wonderfully relaxing therapy was originally used by women to keep their hair thick and healthy.

The upper back, neck and shoulders are the most vulnerable areas for stress so this is where the massage begins. From there the practitioner moves on to the head and scalp, and then the face. The whole session usually lasts around 30 minutes.

MANUAL LYMPHATIC DRAINAGE

This deeply relaxing technique works on the autonomic nervous system, which controls our involuntary impulses such as breathing and stimulates the lymphatic system, the body's waste disposal system.

It was developed in France in the 1930s by Dr. Emil Vodder and his wife Estrid when he noticed that people with chronic catarrhal and sinus infections tended to have lumpy, swollen glands. Contrary to medical practice at that time, he began to work with the lymph nodes. It is now thought that this kind of massage can heal scar tissue, burns and edema (or swelling).

When we are stressed the lymphatic system can become sluggish, which impairs its ability to get rid of the continual influx of the stress hormones, adrenaline and cortisol. An MLD massage helps to shift these toxic hormones and is also wonderfully relaxing.

AROMATHERAPY MASSAGE

"The way to good health is to have an aromatic bath and a scented massage every day." These are not the words of an aromatherapist touting for business, but the beliefs of Hippocrates, the father of modern medicine, writing in the 4th century BC. The term aromatherapy, meaning "treatment using scents" was coined in the 1920s by a French chemist called René Gattefossé, who discovered, while working in his parents' perfumery business, that essential oils had valuable healing properties.

No one really knows how fragrance affects the mind. The most widely held view is that receptors in the nose convert scents into electrical impulses. These are then transmitted to the area of the brain associated with emotional responses, memory, intuition and sex drive. Once there the fragrances directly affect your moods, emotions and mental faculties.

Essential oils also have a pharmacological effect within the body. When applied to the skin in diluted form the molecules in the oils pass through the skin into the bloodstream and are carried throughout the body. They get straight to work on the body tissues and stay longest in those areas of the body which need them most. Certain oils also have an affinity with particular areas of the body: lavender, for example, is extremely effective on the nervous system. (Brazilian research has shown that lavender oils have a sedative effect on the central nervous system, so helping to promote sleep.)

Aromatherapy is used to make you feel better in general. Gentle enough to be used by people of all ages and states of health, its most noticeable benefit is that it de-stresses the mind and body.

There are various ways of using essential oils. The most common and effective method is that used by professional aromatherapists who apply the diluted oils to the skin via a full-body massage. However, your therapist may also advise you to take aromatherapy baths or to burn the oils in a vaporizer at home, as a means of extending the treatment (*see* pp. 209–12). In a few cases, individuals can be allergic to a particular oil, so try them with caution the first time.

REFLEXOLOGY

Reflexology originated in China and Egypt thousands of years ago and has very strong links with acupuncture. Reflexologists work on acupuncture or reflex points on the feet and hands. Our feet are an important but often neglected part of our bodies and their condition has a definite bearing on our general health. Each foot has about 7,000 nerve endings and each of these relates to a specific part of the body. For the reflexologist a person's feet represent a mirror of the body. By stimulating the various reflexes, practitioners increase the flow of energy along the meridians and enhance the body's self-healing abilities.

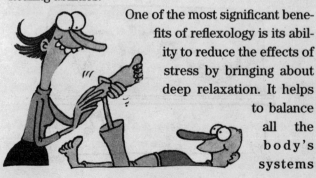

One of the most significant benefits of reflexology is its ability to reduce the effects of stress by bringing about deep relaxation. It helps to balance all the body's systems by stimulating an underactive area and calming an overactive one. Reflexology is a whole-body treatment that works on three levels:

- physiological—resulting in a relaxed and healthy body
- psychological—which creates a calm state of mind and positive outlook by balancing all the body systems
- spiritual—which helps to relax and quiet the emotions.

FLOTATION

An hour in a flotation tank is an effective method of promoting deep relaxation and stress relief.

A flotation tank or cabin is rather like a large covered bath, but the water is only 25 cm/10 in deep.

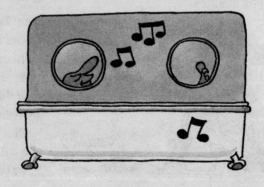

However, the mixture of Epsom and other mineral salts in the water means that your body is completely supported and you cannot help but float, rather like the effect of the Dead Sea.

The water is heated to normal skin temperature—34.2°C/93.56°F—and the salts in the water prevent your skin from drying out.

A session usually lasts an hour. You can opt to have soft music playing, dim light or total darkness. Without the normal stimuli such as light and sound, the brain tends to turn inwards, allowing for an inner awareness. This almost complete sensory deprivation helps lower the heart rate and blood pressure. An hour in a floatation tank is said to be equivalent to five hours of sleep.

HYPNOTHERAPY

This is an effective relaxation therapy for stress- and anxiety-related problems such as phobias and insomnia. The theory behind hypnotherapy is that it helps patients achieve a deeply relaxed state in which they can learn to understand and control their behavior and become more receptive to positive suggestions. Contrary to popular belief, you cannot be hypnotized against your will, nor can you be made to do anything that goes against your usual moral code.

As treatment progresses, self-help techniques

(such as auto-suggestion and self-hypnosis) may be taught to patients for use at home. During the deeply relaxed state, the therapist will introduce positive thoughts for you to focus on each time you find your stress levels rising. You will be given trigger words to use at home. To help you relax even more deeply, the therapist may use guided imagery or visualization of positive scenes and situations (*see* p. 205).

How to Relax at Home

We live in a world of constant activity and one in which we no longer have time to simply relax. Relaxation does not mean, however, sitting like a zombie in front of the TV, nor is it something you cram into ten minutes at the end of your day. It should be something deeper—a temporary state of stillness or meditation in which your usual clutter of thoughts is replaced by a passive awareness.

Studies have shown that practicing relaxation techniques helps to calm people down, reduces the amount of oxygen the body uses, lowers blood lactate levels (high levels of which are linked with anxiety, arousal and high blood pressure), slows the heartbeat and changes brainwave patterns.

LEARN TO MEDITATE

Meditation is the practice of disciplining the mind in

order to quiet mental chatter and transcend outside noise to find a feeling of inner tranquillity and peace.

Although many religions practice some sort of meditation, in itself meditation is not tied to any religious group or creed. In the 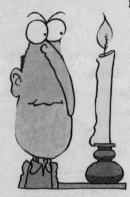 late 1960s and 1970s meditation began to attract the attention of scientists, who found that it helped to lower the metabolic rate and decrease breathing rates. Today it is used in conjunction with conventional medicine, but you don't have to be an expert to experience its benefits.

There are many methods of meditation, but there are two main principles: concentration and overall awareness. To concentrate, you focus on one thing—a beautiful object, your breath, the flame of a candle or a mantra, a simple sound which you repeat to quiet your thoughts. Overall awareness, as practiced by zen devotees, involves simply sitting and being open to the moment, and is quite hard for stressed-out Westerners to learn.

TIPS FOR SUCCESSFUL MEDITATION

- Aim to practice at the same time and same place every day. We are creatures of habit, and establishing a routine will make it easier to stick to.
- Pick a time when you know you will not be disturbed (the best practice times are at the beginning and end of the day).
- Ensure that the room is well ventilated, comfortable, warm and private, and above all peaceful. Burn an incense stick, if you wish.
- Wear loose, comfortable clothing; no tight belts, no shoes.
- Check your posture. Don't attempt to meditate lying down or you'll fall asleep. Sit in a comfortable, straight-backed chair, with your feet flat on the floor and resting your palms on your thighs. Your head should be upright and you should be looking straight ahead.
- Place a clock close by so that you can keep an eye on the time. Remember to turn off the alarm clock. Take the phone off the hook.

Practiced for 20 minutes a day, meditation will energize you, improve your concentration, health and general wellbeing.

MEDITATION TECHNIQUES

Counting the breath. This method involves counting your exhalations. Buddhist practitioners count to ten exhalations, while other disciplines count to four.

Mantra. Repeating a phrase or word over and over again. Some schools believe that what you say is important, but many experts say you can choose any phrase as long as it's repeated aloud. The most popular mantra is the sound Om. You could also try using the sounds Ah, Hum or a combination of the two: Om-Ah. What's more, your mantra can be recited anywhere, any time—while walking the dog or relaxing in the bath—and not just when you are sitting in the meditative position.

Mindfulness. Based on the ancient Buddhist practice *vipassana* (insight) this technique helps you to cultivate a heightened state of awareness. First focus on the rims of your nostrils as your breath goes in and out. Next concentrate on "watching" your thoughts as they rise like bubbles, and observe them without judgment.

BREATHING MEDITATION

This Buddhist practice is deeply relaxing. The aim is to "empty" your mind and focus solely on your breathing. During meditation trivial annoyances may fill up the empty space you have created. Your mind may start to wander and you may even forget where you are in your meditation. When this happens calmly return your attention back to your practice. Distractions are part and parcel of meditation. Don't try to force yourself to concentrate. That would not be relaxing and you will probably end up feeling more frustrated than when you began.

- Before starting, just sit for a minute or so until you feel calm and your breathing feels slow and regular. Close your eyes. Relax your body, feel your weight sinking down towards the floor, and feel any tension melt away.
- Become aware of your breath. At the end of your out breath say "one." Count at the end of each breath up to ten. Repeat for five minutes.
- Now mark each breath at the beginning. Count up to ten and repeat for five minutes.

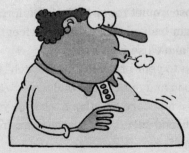

- Now focus on your breathing without counting for five minutes.
- Now focus on the part of your nose where you can feel the cold air meeting the warm. Remain focused in this way for five minutes.
- When you have finished, slowly open your eyes, take in your surroundings, and wait for a couple of minutes before standing up, to avoid dizziness.

EDMUND JACOBSON'S PROGRESSIVE RELAXATION

If you have never practiced any sort of relaxation or meditation technique before this is a good place to start as you tend to get good results every time.

It takes about 15 minutes and should ideally be done twice a day. With each practice you will find that you enter a progressively deeper state of relaxation. (*Note:* allow around ten seconds for each step.)

- Choose a quiet room. Sit in a comfortable straight-backed chair, with your feet flat on the floor and close your eyes.
- Listen to your breathing and "watch" the air come in and out of your body.
- Take a few deep breaths. Each time you exhale slowly and silently repeat the word "relax" to yourself.

- Focus on your face. Feel tension in your face or eyes, jaw or tongue. Make a mental picture of that tension, then imagine the tension disappearing and everything becoming relaxed and limp.
- Feel your face, jaw, eyes and then your tongue becoming relaxed, and as they do so feel a wave of relaxation spreading throughout your body.
- Squeeze all the muscles in your face and eyes as tight as you can. Then let go and feel the relaxation seep around your body.
- Now apply the same instruction to every part of your body: head, neck, shoulders, upper back, arms, hands, mid- and lower back, abdomen, thighs, calves, ankles, feet, and toes.
- When you have covered your entire body sit quietly for about five minutes.
- Now let your eyelids become lighter and give yourself a minute or so before opening your eyes.
- Open your eyes.

AUTOGENIC TRAINING

Psychiatrist Johannes Schultz noted that when you are deeply relaxed your body feels heavy. He also found that just imagining your arms and legs becoming heavy sent a message to your muscles to relax and let go. Based on these observations he developed this simple and highly effective stress-reduction technique.

Give yourself at least ten minutes to complete this exercise.

- Dress in warm comfortable clothing and lie down with a small pillow placed under your head and another under your knees.
- Rest your hands on your stomach, then calmly and slowly inhale for a count of three; feel your stomach rising. Exhale through your mouth for a count of five. Repeat 15 times.
  - Now focus on your dominant arm. Visualize it becoming heavy. Then say to yourself, "My arm is getting heavy." Focus on its weight for 10 to 15 seconds. Feel it sinking into your stomach. Repeat twice more.
- Do the same with your other arm, then each leg in turn, and then return to the original arm.
- Repeat the sequence, but this time say to yourself, "My arm is getting warm." Repeat for the whole of your body.

- Now focus on your forehead and say to yourself, "My forehead feels cool."
- Remain focused on your forehead for a minute then say to yourself, "I feel refreshed and relaxed."

VISUALIZE RELAXING IMAGES

This technique will help to banish tension.

- Lie down in a quiet place and close your eyes.
- Mentally sweep through your body and relax tense muscles.
- Picture an image that uses all your senses (sight, hearing, smell, touch and taste). For example, imagine a white beach fringed with palm trees bent so low their fronds gently stroke the sand. See the clear blue-green water stretching out to the horizon and cloudless azure-blue sky. Hear the surf breaking on the shore. Feel the warm sand between your toes and the warm water bathing your feet as you walk along the water's edge. Smell and taste the salt as it is carried in the warm air.
- Now think of a short, positive statement that affirms the fact that you can relax at will, for example, "My mind is relaxed," "I'm letting go of all stress," "I feel calm and relaxed."

BREATHE TO BEAT STRESS

Stop and listen to your breathing. Is each breath quick and shallow or long and slow? Is your breath in your upper chest or down in your abdomen?

Most people use only half of their lung capacity, and breathe with their chest and not their diaphragm. The diaphragm is a thin, dome-shaped sheet of muscle separating the lungs from the liver and upper part of the abdomen. When you inhale properly your diaphragm contracts and pushes the dome down and your stomach out, and the lungs expand to take up the space left by the diaphragm dropping.

This is a mechanism that we are born with. But by the time we become adults we have forgotten how to breathe with our diaphragm and tend to use our chest instead. Relearning how to breathe with your diaphragm will help your body to work better.

The way you breathe also reflects your emotional state. When you are anxious or stressed, your breathing becomes rapid and shallow. When you are happy, your breathing is naturally slower and deeper.

FULL BREATHING

1. Lie on a rug on the floor or on a firm bed with your hands resting on your abdomen above your navel. (If you suffer from back problems it

may be helpful either to roll up a towel and place it under your lower back or bend your knees while keeping your feet on the floor, so you create a triangle.)

2. Close your eyes and inhale deeply and slowly, so that your hands are lifted slightly towards the ceiling. Don't force the breath.

3. Exhale slowly applying a light pressure on your abdomen to encourage full elimination.

Repeat 15 times. After completing this exercise, wait a few moments before getting up to avoid dizziness.

CHECK YOUR BREATHING

Are you breathing with your diaphragm?

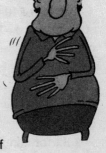

- Lie on your back on the floor.
- Place one hand on your stomach and the other on your chest.
- Focus on your hands and notice which hand rises first. If your chest moves first, you are not breathing with your diaphragm and making full use of your lung capacity.

ALTERNATE NOSTRIL BREATHING

- Wearing loose clothing, sit comfortably in a straight-backed chair or cross-legged on the floor.
- Shut your eyes, take deep breaths in and out and focus on your breathing.
- Close your right nostril with your right thumb. Exhale through the left and inhale to a count of four.
- Close the left nostril with the ring finger and little finger of your right hand. Hold your breath for a count of 16.
- Release your right nostril and exhale fully through a count of eight.
- Keeping your left nostril closed, inhale through the right to a count of four.
- Close both nostrils and hold your breath to a count of 16.
- Release the left nostril and exhale to a count of eight.

Repeat this sequence 10 times daily. When exhaling, try to empty your lungs completely.

- Sit for minute or two breathing regularly to allow the exercise to work fully.

If you start to feel dizzy, rest for a while, open your eyes and breathe normally. Continue as soon as you feel comfortable. Don't strain to control your breathing.

AROMATHERAPY

An aromatherapy massage is a wonderful way to relax and de-stress (*see* p. 191). But there are also a number of ways in which to benefit from this aromatic therapy at home when you don't have a masseur on hand.

BATHS

A long soak in an aromatic bath is a wonderful way to unwind at the end of a stressful day. Oils can be used to improve your mood, to help you relax or to stimu-

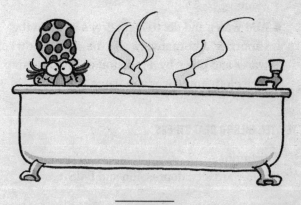

late your body. Essential oils don't dissolve but form a thin layer on the surface. The heat of the water releases the scent and helps them to be absorbed by the skin.

- Fill the bath with warm water, then four to eight drops of oil and agitate the water to disperse. Don't add the oil while you are running your bath or much of the aromatic vapor will evaporate before you get in.
- If you have dry skin, try mixing the essential oil with a base oil such as sweet almond, sunflower or hazelnut.

VAPORIZERS

These are a wonderful way to scent a room and enhance your mood.

- Add water and six to eight drops of oil to the vaporizer. Alternatively, add the oil to a bowl of water and place by a radiator, or on to a damp face cloth hung over a radiator.

TOP TEN OILS TO BEAT STRESS

Bergamot
Use for: anxiety, depression and PMS

Caution: avoid using oil shortly before exposing your skin to sunlight as it may cause you to go red or burn

Roman chamomile
Use for: inflamed skin conditions, aches and pains, PMS, headaches, insomnia, nervous tension
Caution: avoid during pregnancy

Clary sage
Use for: high blood pressure, depression, migraine, insomnia, nervous tension
Caution: avoid during pregnancy

Geranium
Use for: poor circulation and nervous tension
Caution: none

Lavender
Use for: respiratory problems, muscular aches and pains, headaches, depression, insomnia, nervous tension
Caution: none

Neroli
Use for: skin care, palpitations, PMS, depression and stress-related conditions
Caution: none

Rose otto
Use for: respiratory problems, insomnia, headache, PMS, nervous tension
Caution: avoid during pregnancy

Rosemary
Use for: respiratory problems, aches and pains, poor circulation, headaches, mental fatigue, depression and nervous exhaustion
Caution: avoid during pregnancy

Sandalwood
Use for: insomnia, PMS, depression and other stress-related conditions
Caution: none

Ylang ylang
Use for: high blood pressure, palpitations, depression, insomnia, nervous tension
Caution: none

LEARN HOW TO GROUND YOURSELF

Feelings of stress and high anxiety are often accompanied by a sense of weightlessness; a feeling that our feet are not quite on the ground.

The following exercise will help to relax you

before any nerve-racking event and should dispel feelings of anxiety and panic.

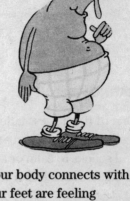

- Draw an imaginary circle on the floor and step into it. Stand comfortably, so that your body weight is fully supported.
- Breathe deeply and tune into the inflow and out-flow. Now focus on your navel and relax.
- Become aware of how your body connects with the earth. Notice that your feet are feeling heavy. Visualize weights attached to the soles of your feet, anchors or sandbags, perhaps, or the roots of a tree. Now imagine letting those weights or roots sink into the floor, through the floorboards and right down into the center of the earth. Breathing deeply and easily, spend a few moments experiencing that feeling of being connected with the center of the earth, noticing how strong and powerful you feel.

A Stress-free Lifestyle

EATING WELL

One of the biggest influences on our minds and bodies is our diet. Eating sensible, well-balanced meals and snacks to calm or energize us throughout the day makes it much easier for us to counteract the effects of stress.

HOW STRESSFUL IS YOUR DIET?

Run down the checklist of bad habits below and make a note of how many you are guilty of. If you score more than three it's time to start changing your eating habits.

Do you:

- eat too many high-sugar or fatty snacks?
- drink excessive amounts of coffee to keep you going?
- drink alcohol for relaxation or comfort?
- grab any old snack or quick meal on the run?

SNACK ATTACK

Resist the temptation to snack on cookies and chocolates and endless cups of coffee. Eat three of the following snacks a day to help keep that mid-afternoon slump at bay:

- low-fat, low-sugar fruit yogurt or fromage frais
- grapes, bananas, kiwi fruit, apples or pears
- raw celery, carrot, cauliflower, radish or cucumber
- pumpkin and sunflower seeds, unsalted
- dried figs and apricots
- almonds and walnuts, unsalted
- low-salt whole-wheat biscuits spread with a little low-fat cream cheese
- whole-wheat pita with salad
- fruit (or plain) muffin

- rely on take-out and convenience foods?
- bolt down your food?
- eat irregularly or late at night?
- eat at your desk or slumped in a chair?
- eat more than you need to because you haven't eaten anything else for hours?

If you develop the following good habits your stress levels should fall dramatically:

- Eat three meals a day: don't skip breakfast—

this is the most important meal of the day and will help keep your blood-sugar levels steady and sustain your energy. Regular meals re-energize the mind and body.

- Stop and eat: even if it's only for half an hour.

Research shows that mealtimes are a time of relaxation. If you have to eat in the office try to eat at another desk, so that you have a break from the source of your stress.

- Eat slowly: chew food well to aid digestion. Give yourself a few minutes after you have finished eating to allow your stomach to start the digestive process.
- Eat fresh food: this will provide essential vitamins and minerals that your body needs more than ever when you are stressed.
- Don't overeat: digesting a huge meal will rob you of energy.
- Eat regular snacks: these help to curb sugar cravings but don't use them as a substitute for regular meals.
- Don't eat late at night, and wait at least three hours between your meal and bedtime to allow your body time to digest your food properly.
- Don't eat if you are angry, upset or agitated:

practice one of the relaxation techniques on
pp. 175–85, or go for a walk and then eat.

EAT TO BEAT STRESS

The best defense against destructive stress is a
healthy body and nutritious diet.

- Eat two or more servings per day of vitamin-
  rich foods, such as citrus fruits and dark green
  leafy vegetables.
- Eat foods rich in vitamin A and folic acid—dark
  green or orange vegetables and orange juice.
- Eat plenty of whole, unprocessed foods such as
  wholegrain breads and cereals, dried beans and
  peas, fresh fruit and vegetables and low-fat milk.
- Eat iron-rich foods such as dried beans and
  peas and leafy green vegetables.
- Zinc and magnesium are great stress-busters
  and are found in seafood, dried beans and
  whole grains.
- Cut out refined sugars, caffeine and sodium.
- Drink plenty of water (at least four glasses a
  day) to flush out waste matter.
- Protein, fat and carbohydrates are speedily
  used up during periods of stress. Carbohydrates
  are particularly important as they provide
  steady amounts of energy throughout the day.

AVOID STRESS-AGGRAVATING FOODS

CAFFEINE

Cut back on: coffee, tea, and cola drinks. Drink no more than two cups a day. Caffeine is also in many drug preparations such as aspirin.

Effects: boosts adrenaline release.

Try to: switch to herbal teas.

ALCOHOL

Cut back on: overdoing it!

Effects: boosts adrenaline release.

Try to: avoid drinking when you feel stressed out.

SUGAR

Cut back on: sugary desserts, cakes and sweets.

Effects: boosts adrenaline release.

Try to: switch to fresh fruit for dessert.

SALT

Cut back on: adding salt to food, salty snacks and foods such as olives, pickles, sauces and stock cubes.

Effects: raises blood pressure and depletes your adrenal glands.

Try to: switch to fresh fruit snacks. Use more spices to replace salt when you are cooking.

HERBAL HELP FOR STRESS

The following herbs are available in supplements from pharmacies and health food stores. Take according to the manufacturers' instructions:

- Ginseng
- Valerian
- Chamomile
- Kava Kava
- St. John's Wort or hypericum

MEAT, FISH AND DAIRY PRODUCTS

Cut back on: saturated fat in dairy products, animal and vegetable fat, coconut oil, palm oil, hard margarine and cookies, cakes and desserts.

Effects: can change the body's sodium balance, leading to weak muscles and nervousness.

Try to: switch to skimmed milk, low-fat margarine, unprocessed live yogurt. Grill, roast or steam meat, eat more legumes and vegetables, replace meat with fish.

GET FIT

Exercise is an important part of stress management.

It provides emotional and mental relief, and it is the best way to get rid of the barrage of hormones flowing around our body whenever the typical stress fight-or-flight response is triggered.

Three sessions a week of aerobic exercise lasting around 20–30 minutes will help to get you fit, which will, in turn, increase your sense of wellbeing. Regular exercise will also improve the quality of your sleep, which is vital if your body is to cope well with stress.

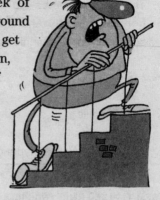

- Walking, jogging and swimming are ideal forms of aerobic exercise.
- Research has shown that the effects of exercise are cumulative and lots of small sessions are as useful as an hour in the gym.

Try to:
- take a walk during your lunch hour
- walk to stores instead of taking the car
- get off the bus a few stops from your destination and walk the rest of the way
- use the stairs instead of an elevator.

LEARN YOGA

This 2000-year-old practice is an ideal method of dealing with modern stresses. Yoga philosophy believes that life's challenges can be solved by building up inner strength and character.

Yoga is a combination of gentle movement and deep stretches, breathing exercises, visualization and meditation techniques which train the mind to focus. Regular practice will not only create a well-toned body, it will also help to produce inner calm and tranquillity, strength and clarity of mind.

TAKE UP T'AI CHI

T'ai chi, also known as *t'ai chi chu'an*, is an ancient Chinese discipline based on the belief that "chi" energy or life force flowing freely is essential for good health. T'ai chi combines movement and meditation.

The flowing, dance-like exercises of t'ai chi strengthen your inner energy, while deep breathing and soothing imagery calm your mind. It is an ideal form of exercise for people of all ages and fitness levels because the movements do not require any strength or exertion. The sequences work on nearly every muscle and joint, improving body control.

PRACTICE PILATES

Developed by Joseph Pilates, a prisoner of war who came up with the technique to improve the health of his fellow inmates, Pilates concentrates on elongating and straightening the body. The combination of gentle stretches and breath control helps to keep the body strong, supple and flexible, and promotes deep relaxation, releasing stress and tension.

QUIT SMOKING

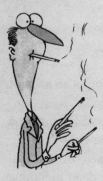

Many smoking-related diseases are also stress-related, and research has shown that smoking when you are stressed exacerbates the stress response. This could be because when we are stressed we breathe more quickly and rapidly, which enables more smoke to enter the lungs than when we are relaxed.

BOOST YOUR SELF-ESTEEM

The thoughts, feelings and beliefs you hold about yourself are all interdependent, and the manner in which you "speak" to yourself can make a dramatic difference to your self-esteem.

If, for the most part, your self-talk is negative and critical, you will start to feel increasingly worthless and miserable. Repeating affirmations is a good way to turn this negative speak around. Try one of the following:

- I am deserving.
- I am worthwhile.
- I accept myself completely.
- I allow myself to be happy now.
- I am calm, confident and in control.
- With each day that passes I am becoming increasingly confident.
- I am becoming a more relaxed person.
- I am banishing inappropriate negative beliefs from my mind.

You can repeat them out loud when you're on your own, or quietly, in your head, when faced with difficult or threatening situations.

ARE YOU YOUR OWN WORST ENEMY?

If you have grown up with poor self-esteem you may feel unworthy of the good things that life has to offer, or you won't want to go after brilliant jobs because you are afraid of failure. It may be that by doing this you are subconsciously sabotaging your own chance of happiness and success.

The idea that we may be responsible for our own failure can be difficult to accept, especially if we believe that we are doing the best we can. After all, what fool would deliberately set out to destroy their chances of getting their dream job or house?

Self-sabotage occurs in various ways—it may be emotional, financial or physical—through developing certain habits that hold you back, says Nancy Go, the author of *Slay Your Own Dragons* (Sheldon Press). Some are more obvious than others:

- spending so much time on a job application that you "accidentally" miss the deadline.
- developing travel anxieties so that it limits your range of opportunities.
- being so critical or difficult in relationships that you drive your partner away.

Try answering the questions on page 225 to see if you fit into this category.

HOW TO STOP SABOTAGING YOUR LIFE:

- Take time to be on your own and relax. Don't be afraid of the feelings that may occur. By learning how to face them head-on you'll be better equipped to deal with them.

ARE YOU SABOTAGING YOUR LIFE?

Read through the following list. How many statements do you agree with?

- I am regularly late for appointments.
- I tend to worry more about others than about myself.
- I tend to procrastinate.
- I'm a perfectionist.
- I'm indecisive.
- I always get involved with the wrong type of partner.
- I often think that my life would be better if only I were more intelligent/better-looking/taller/thinner.
- I never seem to have time to do the things that are important to me.
- I tend to live in the past or the future rather than focusing on today.
- I am always in debt.
- I often put myself down.

If you agree with more than five of the above, it's time you took a good look at your life to try and discover why you are so intent on destroying your chances of happiness.

- Break out of self-destructive habits. Learn how to spot the triggers, feelings and ways of behavior that are setting you up for failure and find new ways to behave. But keep it simple, don't replace one type of self-defeating behavior with another.
- Visualizing the result you want will help you to achieve it. Sit in a relaxed position and then imagine yourself succeeding at a job interview, passing your driving test, or meeting someone nice at a party.
- Stop blaming yourself when things go wrong. We all make mistakes. Simply accept that you did your best—then let it go. No one is perfect so don't dwell on past mistakes.
- Listen to your inner voice and challenge destructive thoughts. If you find yourself thinking, "there's no point taking my driving test because I will only fail," force yourself to challenge that thought.
- Look after yourself. Decide now to put your physical and emotional health first. If you have been putting off going to the gym because you are too busy, reorganize your life so that taking regular exercise becomes as much a part of your life as brushing your teeth twice a day.
- Be your own best friend. If you don't love and respect yourself, why should anyone else?

EVERYDAY STRESS MANAGEMENT

Banish stress from your life with these simple every-day strategies:

- Use the ring of the telephone or the start-up sound of your computer as your cue to take a few deep relaxing breaths.
- Before each meal, rather than digging straight in, take time to breathe and relax. Stop what you are doing when you eat—try to avoid working lunches.
- Slow down. When you are washing the dishes, cleaning the house or waiting for the photo-copier to warm up, you need to realize that you won't save much time by thinking of all the other tasks you could be doing. Use these "spare" moments to clear your mind and relax.
- Use your journey home from work to adjust from the more frantic pace of work to the more relaxed rhythms of home. Just sit in your car for a few minutes before you enter the house, to allow this shift to occur.
- Pause after completing one task before starting another. Practice mindfulness by doing one job at a time and give it your full attention.
- Take a day off once in a while (not just because

you are ill), and simply enjoy the feeling of not having to do anything in particular.

STOP BEING SO NICE

Every time you make excuses for someone, smooth things over to keep the peace, or to avoid conflict, you are being too nice. It means that you are not expressing your feelings effectively which can lead to a negative backlash of misdirected anger towards yourself or a third party who just happened to get in the way. Here's how to be more assertive:

- Don't rise to the bait or get drawn into conversations that you don't want to have by trying to reason with the other person.
- Move things forward. If the conversation is going around in circles, call a time-out to get the discussion back on a positive track.
- Maintain eye contact. If someone can see your face properly they will know how genuine your feelings are.
- Speak firmly. This does not mean raising your

voice or shouting, but what you say has to be said in a strong enough way to convey what you really mean.

● Repeat yourself. This will ensure that the other person has got the message and will help you to stand your ground.

BE A BETTER DECISION-MAKER

● Do as much research as you can about any decision. Talk with people you trust or get expert advice if necessary. Careful preparation and checking can help to preempt a disaster.

● Look at the future and consider the best- and worst-case scenarios that could arise from your decision: look at the effect it could have on yourself and on everyone concerned.

● Give yourself thinking space. If you feel under pressure, don't agree to a decision immediately. Ask for more time so that you can make a considered choice.

SLEEP IT OFF

Without sleep your body cannot rest and repair itself. So a good night's sleep is essential to stress control. When you are asleep, two distinct patterns alternate throughout the night: deep, dreamless sleep, known as

NREM—non-rapid-eye-movement sleep—and REM—rapid-eye-movement sleep, when you dream.

If you are having trouble sleeping try some of the following an hour or so before bedtime.

- Take a warm bath to help relax you.
- Avoid stimulating drinks such as tea, coffee or cola.
- Have a cup of warm milk. Milk contains tryptophan, the amino acid which triggers the release of the sleep hormone.
- Don't read anything work-related in bed.
- Don't read thrillers or anything so exciting that you won't want to put it down.

KEEP YOUR SLEEP PATTERN IN ORDER

- Allow enough time for sleep and make sure that you go to bed and wake up at about the same time every day.
- Don't go to bed feeling hungry or with a full stomach.
- If you have a bath before bed, dim the lights in the bathroom or, better still, bathe by candlelight.
- Sleep in complete darkness.
- Open your curtains as soon as you wake up.

LEARN TO SEE THE FUNNY SIDE

Stress can rob you of your sense of humor and fun. Research shows that having a good laugh improves 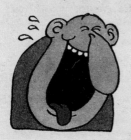 your respiration, lowers blood pressure, exercises your heart muscles and internal organs and builds up your immune system. Laughter helps to lower levels of the stress hormone cortisol and increases the number and the activity of your body's natural killer cells (the white blood cells that fight infection).

If you're having trouble finding humor in everyday life, rent a couple of comedy videos or read a funny book. Then notice your stress and tension fall away.

Best of all, arrange a night out with your funniest, most cheerful friends, and soon you will find yourself laughing about the foibles of your kids, your partner, your boss, or some of the other stresses in your life. Everything has a funny side!